BOOKS AND HOME STUDY COURSES
by Goswami Kriyananda

Books

Spiritual Science of Kriya Yoga
Beginner's Guide to Meditation
Intermediate Guide to Meditation
Advanced Guide to Meditation
The Wisdom and Way of Astrology
The Bhagavad Gita
The Laws of Karma
Extraordinary Spiritual Potential
Kriya Yoga Upanishad and the Ten Mystical Yoga Upanishads
Pathway to God-Consciousness
Yoga Dictionary of Basic Sanskrit Terms
Yoga Dictionary of Basic Astrological Terms
Beginner's Guide to Meditation, A Talking Book
Beginner's Guide to Meditation, Book-Tape Set
Wisdom & Way of Astrology

Home Study Courses

The Chakras: The Garden of God
Kriology
Sacred Apprenticeship: Guru-Disciple Relationship
Philosophy and Methodology of Kriya Yoga
Establishing a Firm Foundation for Your Spiritual Life
The Yoga Sutras of Patanjali
Hatha Yoga Teacher Training & Certification Home Study

In French

La Science Spirituelle du Kriya Yoga
Guide Pratique de Méditation
Astrologie, voie de Sagesse
Les Lois du Karma
Le Kriya Bindu

In Spanish

Su Primer Guía de Meditación

In Italian

La scienza spirituale delle yoga di Kriya
E.S.P.: tuoi eccezionali poteri spirituali
Astrology: via e saggezza

In Dutch

Kriya Yoga: Werk en Oefenboek

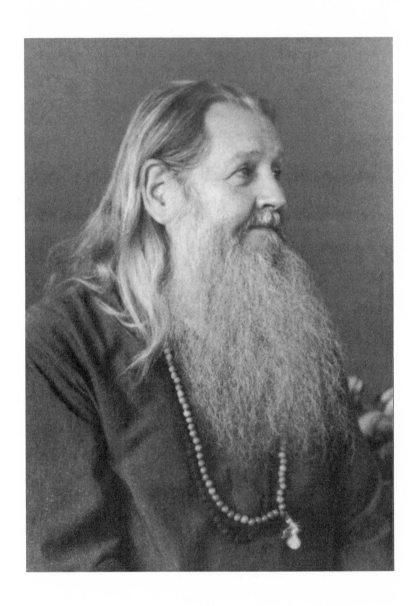

A Yoga Dictionary
of Basic Sanskrit Terms

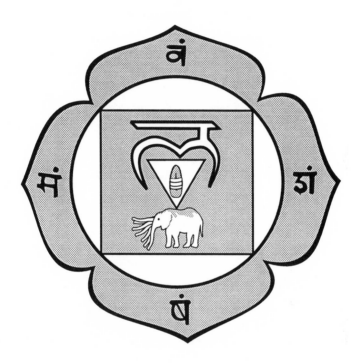

Goswami Kriyananda

The Temple of Kriya Yoga

· Chicago ·

ISBN: 0-929522-02-8

Published by:
        The Temple of Kriya Yoga
        2414 N. Kedzie Blvd
        Chicago, IL   60647
        (312) 342-4600

Printed in the United States of America.

INTRODUCTION

The need for a fresh, simple dictionary of basic Sanskrit terms that would meet the demands of the contemporary student as well as the general reader of yoga has long been acknowledged. It is my hope that this small dictionary will fulfill that need. I have added a supplementary section of basic English mystical terms which I feel will be helpful in giving added depth to this dictionary.

Because the field of Hindu philosophy is so vast, an inclusion of all key words would rapidly turn this dictionary into several books. Thus, I have had to limit the key words. If you feel some key words were left out, please write me in care of the Temple of Kriya Yoga, and they will be included in the next edition.

In using this dictionary please keep in mind a few basic points:

1. I have not made a distinction between long and short vowels in Sanskrit words.
2. I have hyphenated some Sanskrit words for ease of pronunciation.
3. I have also pluralized some Sanskrit words with an English 's.'
4. Finally, the Sanskrit letter 'v' is pronounced like an English 'w.' Thus, 'sattva' is pronounced as if it were spelled 'sattwa.'

For correct Sanskrit spelling, pluralizing, special markings, and correct euphonic rules, refer to a basic Sanskrit grammar.

Yours in the Dharma,

Goswami Kriyananda

A
The first letter of the Sanskrit alphabet. In Sanskrit, all the vowels come together followed by all the consonants. '*A*' means 'that from which all else is borne.'

ABHINIVESHA
Most often refers to the desire for bodily life, or the thirst for physical life. It is one of the five key causes for malcontentment. (See *kleshas*.) This desire for physical bodily existence springs from ignorance because a person wrongly identifies himself/herself with the body, and therefore the survival instinct of the physical body overrides higher instincts. Often referred to as *possessiveness*.

ABHYANTARA-BAHYA-STAMAHA-VRITTI
Extended four-phase motion breath.

ABHYASA
Means 'practice.' It is one of the fundamental requirements for the spiritual life. The other fundamental requirement is dispassion. (See *vairagya*.) Without these two fundamentals, success in the spiritual life is not possible.

ACHARYA
A teacher who lives his philosophy.

ADHI
A prefix meaning 'superior' or 'over.' The three most important nouns using this prefix are:

1. *Adhy-atma* and its adjectival form, adhyatmika - which refers to afflictions and/or hindrances which arise or manifest from one's own self.
2. *Adhi-daiva* and its adjectival form, adhidaivika - which refers to afflictions and/or hindrances which arise or manifest from one's own planetary forces. (See *deva*).
3. *Adhi-bhuta* and it adjectival form, adhibautika - which refers to afflictions and/or hindrances which arise or manifest from other earth life-forms.

Of course, all hindrances and all afflictions always arise because of one's own karma.

ADHIKARA
The 'illumination' in the mind of the giver, given along with a sacred technique or sacred knowledge

ADHI-SHESHA
(See *ananta.*)

ADHOBASTI
A cleansing technique used on the colon.

ADITYA(S)
The sons of Aditi who is the Vedic goddess of ether (space). She is the personification of the various aspects of solar energy. Her name means 'unlimited,' which is the unbounded realm beyond the earth, sky, and heaven. Above the manifested four lower chakras, Aditi represents cosmic energy.

The Shatapatha Brahmana states that the twelve sons of Aditi represent each of the twelve zodiacal signs with its manifesting energies and occult secrets. All the Adityas are aspects of light and are collectively regarded as one, called the Aditya—the Sun. All the worlds are attached to the Aditya by a thread: like beads on a necklace. The Sun is one of the six doors to the impersonal Sri Brahman. At the dissolution of the world, the Adityas will appear as twelve Suns; hence, the Sun is said to be twelve-souled. The Adityas are: Vishnu, Shakra, Aryaman, Dhuti, Tvastri, Pusan, Vivasvat, Savitri, Mitra, Varuna, Amsha and Bhaga.

Aditya also means a person who practices celibacy until the age of 48.

ADYANTARA
Internal pranayama.

AGNI (SRI)
The deva of fire. In Vedic times Sri Agni was most suitable to act as the messenger to the higher states of consciousness. Fire or kriya-kundalini was the predominating feature of the sacrifice. The fire on the external altar always rose and thus became the exoteric symbol of the internal fire. Owing to his nature, Sri Agni and the other devas were less anthropomorphically described than metaphorically related.

Sri Agni is the priest of the devas as well as the deva of the priest. Sri Deva had 49 sons (7 X 7), symbolic of the 49 fires. Sri Agni's ultimate aspect is the subterranean fire which will finally emerge from the cavity of the Saturn chakra and dissolve the lower states of consciousness in man, replenishing them in phoenix fashion with higher states of consciousness.

AGNI PRASANA
The fire-breath.

AGNISARA DHAUTI
Fire stomach cleaning.

AHAM BRAHMASMI
A yogic affirmation meaning, 'I am the creative principle.'

AHAMKARA
Means 'I-maker.' It commonly refers to that which applies to the bundle of traits embracing the body and mind, and referred to as 'myself.' It is often used to express one's own ego, or the principle of individuation. In yoga we stress the need to move from ego-awareness to (True) Self-awareness.

AHAMKARA MUDRA
A mudra made by joining the thumb at the center of the index finger.

AHIMSA
Means 'non-violence.' It is the mystical undertaking to live without causing injury to others, or self, and at the same time to act in such a way as to cause others, (and self), happiness. This non-violence relates to their bodies, thoughts, emotions, feelings and possessions. Non-violence must be practiced in deed, speech and thought.

AJAPA MANTRA
The subconscious and automatic repetition of the *hamsa* mantra. In this mantra, the *ham* mantra sound relates to the out-going breath, and the *sa* mantra sound relates to the in-going breath. This mantra is a creative mantra and thus gives physical creative power to earthlings. It is the opposite of the *hong-sau* mantra in which the *hong* mantra relates to the in-breath, and thus bestows spiritual powers to the earthling.

AJNA CHAKRA

The Sun center chakra existing at the root of the nose between the eyebrows. This chakra is the spiritual heart of the seeker. It is the place of the 'sixth sense,' or intuition. It has two petals, one having on it the sound 'HA,' and the other having on it the sound 'KSHA.' The practice of formless meditation leads to hearing the voice of the Inner Guru (clairaudience). It also leads to awareness of the astral realms wherein Lord Indra (King of the astral gods) resides. The bija mantra for this chakra is 'OM.'

AKARNA DHANURA

The shooting-bow pose.

AKASHA

Today it means *ether*, the first of the most subtle of the five elements. The word means 'luminous,' but rapidly came to mean 'space.' It was used as a symbol of the Higher Self, which was more radiant than 10,000 Suns. Traditionally, ether exists in the Mercury chakra, in the throat area. There are historically five ethers. These five ethers are:

The ether without qualities,
The supreme ether,
The great ether,
The ether of truth,
The solar ether.

Each ether is a radiant space from which an inner experience manifests. Through merging with these five radiant experiences which act as stepping stones, the mystic merges with the Reality.

ALAMBASA

A celestial woman born of Kashyapa. She functions symbolically as a temptress, which relates to the secondary nadi called *alambasa*.

ALINGA

That which has no characters nor any attributes. Thus it relates to the Formless Reality. It is a symbol for the Parama-Vishnu of the Gita, or the Parama-Shiva of the yogis, or the Parama-Brahman of the Upanishads.

ALLAHABAD

The Islamic name of one of the seven sacred cities of the Hindus situated at the confluence of the Ganges, the Jamuna (Yamuna), and the mythical subterranean river called Sarasvati. In the ancient days this city was called Prayaga: the place of sacrifice where Lord Brahman performed the horse sacrifice. It is one of the internal tirthas.

ANAHATA CHAKRA
The mass-energy center located at the heart level. In mystical terms it is called the Venus center. It has 12 petals, and each petal has engraved on it a letter of the Sanskrit alphabet. This chakra bears the first consonant 'K.' The other letters are: KH, G, GH, N, CH, CHH, J, JH, N, T, and TH. The first 'N' is guttural. The second 'N' is palatal. The 'T' and the 'TH' are both cerebrals. This chakra contains the air element or tattva. Right below this chakra is a very small, eight-petalled chakra called *upa-anahata chakra*. According to some mystics, it contains the pain of all human suffering. One should not meditate upon this upa-chakra.

ANANDA
Means 'bliss,' which is one of the attributes of pure consciousness which makes up the basic Reality. As the mystic ascends his astral spine, he enters into an inner state called, 'ananda-maya-kosha,' and there experiences pure bliss.

ANANDA MAYA KOSHA
The bliss sheath. (See *kosha*.)

ANANDA SAMADHI
The fifth level of samadhi in which bliss is felt after the transcending of all objective 'realities.'

ANANTA
The word means 'endless' or 'eternity.' It is the name of the great coiled serpent upon which Lord Vishnu reclines during the Night of Brahma. In the deeper symbolism, the mystic must consistently remind himself that he is not to be ruled by time, and thus keeps in his mind and realizes that the spiritual task of reaching the Realization of Reality will take an infinite amount of patience and endless practice. This serpent-couch is symbolized by a seven-headed, or a 1000-headed serpent called adhi-shesha. *Shesha* means 'remainder,' for it is what remains after the Day of Brahma.

ANATMA.
The non-self, which is the total universe of manifestation.

ANGAS
The steps or phases of yoga practice, often referred to as the 'limbs of yoga.' In some texts there are four stages, in other texts there are 15 stages. However, in classical yoga, in *Patanjali's Yoga Sutras*, there are eight stages. These are:

> Self-discipline or the abstinences: *yama*
> Self-restraint or the observances: *niyama*
> The meditative postures: *asana*
> Breath control: *pranayama*
> Sense withdrawal: *pratyahara*
> Concentration: *dharana*
> Meditation: *dhyana*
> Contemplation: samadhi.

The first four are considered as 'outer or gross' stages, whereas, the last four are considered 'inner or subtle' stages.

ANGIRAS
A famous rishi or sage associated with the kriya kundalini fire ritual. He is often referred to by other sages as their ancient father. Angiras is regarded as the first sacrificer and initiator of the sacred fire ritual. Angiras is the one who sought to enlighten mankind with his transcendental teachings and therefore is associated with light and all luminous objects. His identification is with the planet Jupiter, called *Guru* in Sanskrit. He is also associated with one of the key stars in the constellation of Ursa Major.

ANTAH-KARANA
The complete, four-fold instrument of the mind which functions between the Self (Atma) and the physical body. This internal mechanism has four major functions:

1. That which gives identity to the concept of oneself (aham-kara).
2. That which gives an evaluation or an interpretation (correctly or incorrectly) to the sensations and ideas (buddhi).
3. That which compares or classifies ideas and reflects on them (manas).
4. That which collects and stores these sensations and ideas (chitta). The chitta is often referred to as the 'lower mind.'

ANU-LOMA
Regulated nadi-breath.

ANU-LOMA VI-LOMA
Regulated counter current nadi breathing.

ANUSVARA
Anuswara is the *bindu*, or fading away of AUMM, a soundless final 1/2 mora.

APANA
One of the ten vital breaths in Sanskrit called vayus. These are forces of nature which vitalize the various parts of the physical as well as the astral body through the various chakras. Apana as one of the vital breaths is regarded as very holy and the second most important. It is the downward current which relates to and circulates through the Saturn chakra and flushes out the residues of karmic matter in the astral body. Its color is red or red-orange.

APARI-GRAHA
Non-greed or greedlessness. It is the fifth category of the abstinences. It is the attitudinal abandonment of possession. However, it is often wrongly interpreted as abandonment of all possessions. Its true meaning is, not to be attached to possessions, and to possess only that which is truly necessary. On an esoteric level, it means that there is a correct way of taking, holding and using all possessions whether it be clothing, books, food or shelter. The key aim is to be at peace with the objects of this world, and thus with this world. It assists in quieting and focusing the mind. Patanjali states that the mastery of non-greed gives you the power to reveal the meaning and reason of a birth (your own or others).

APAROSH ANUBHUTI
Direct perception. The Realization of God or of the Higher Self cannot be attained by knowledge, inference, nor by other's testament. The Realization of Reality can only be attained by direct perception.

ARANYAKA
The Forest Teachings written by and for those sages who were living in the forests. They precede the Upanishads in the Vedas.

ARDHA-BHUJANGA
The half-cobra pose.

ARDHA-CHANDRA
The half-Moon pose.

ARDHA-MATRA
This term refers to a half-beat found in most mantras. This last half of a short beat is indicated by a dot above the 'm.' Many times it is indicated by just using the letter 'm,' as in Aum, or the bija seed sounds: yam, lam, vam, etc. It has the sound of 'ng' as in sing. The ardha-matra means that the lips should be closed before the letter of the alphabet is sounded. It has a deeper esoteric meaning as related in the mystical yoga Upanishads.

ARDHA-MATSYA-INDRA
The half-spinal twist pose.

ARDHA-SALABHA
The half-locust pose.

ARJUNA
The hero of the Gita, and the disciple of Donacharya. He is symbolically each earthling, who can and will overcome negative and 'evil,' if he chooses Reality to guide his life. In this text the Reality is symbolized as Lord Krishna.

ASAM-PRAJNA SAMADHI
A state of samadhi without seed, which is to say a state which is beyond all perception of content.

ASAN(A)
A yogic posture held to induce various mind states and/or to release spiritual energies. A posture to be a yoga posture must be enjoyable and steady. Asan is not just a physical posture, but also a mental pose, i.e., a correct attitude: peacefulness, quietude. Patanjali does not give a preference to any asan. However, historically there are 84 such postures used in hatha yoga. The hatha postures, including the lotus pose, are meant to be held for only a few seconds. Esoterically, asans refer only to the meditative postures. The meditative poses, excluding the lotus pose, are meant to be held for long periods of time. There are eight meditative poses. The outstanding ones are:

The easy pose: *sukhasan*
The adept's pose: *siddhasan*
The cow pose: *gomukhasan*
The lightening bolt pose: *virasana*
The prosperous pose: *swatikasana*
The lotus pose: *padmasana*.

ASAT

Not being, or non-being. According to the Yoga-Sankhya philosophy, Being can only arise from Being. This is a rejection of Western theology which holds that creation arose from nothingness.

ASHRAM(A)

The dwelling of a Guru and his closer disciples which is devoted to spiritual practices.

Also, ashrama relates to the four stages in a person's life. Each stage is divided into 20 to 25 years. The first stage is picking up the responsibilities of being a student, and learning as a preparation for adult life. The second stage is picking up the responsibilities of a householder or family person. The third stage is withdrawal from active business and social life, as well as studies relating to the 'inner life.' The fourth and last stage is that of renunciation of all worldly ambitions and worldly desires. A person who reaches this fourth stage is called a sannyasi. It is possible to forego the first three stages and become a sannyasi at any adult age. In short, the first stage gives emphasis to our physical and intellectual development. The second stage gives emphasis to mastering our emotional side. The third stage gives emphasis to higher mental development. The fourth stage emphasizes a blending of the three with a development of a deeper spiritual life.

ASHVIN(S)

The name of two divinities who appear in the sky before dawn in a carriage drawn by horses or by birds. The word *ashvin* means 'possessed of horses.' They are said to be twin stars and thus identified with the astrological constellation of Gemini. They are referred to as the Suns of the sea, meaning the atmosphere, which they regard as an ocean of air whose ultimate shores are earth and heaven.

ASMITA

The state of ego, or of 'I-am-ness.' The awareness one feels that he is a distinct and separate being. Classically, it is the error of confusing that which is seen, with the seer; confusing that which is heard, with the hearer; and confusing that which is known, with the knower, etc.

ASMITA SAMADHI
The sixth level of samadhi.

ASTEYA
Non-stealing. It is the third of the abstinences.

ASURA
Means 'lord' in the earlier Vedic period. The word comes from the root *as*, meaning 'to exist,' or from *ashu*, meaning 'to breathe.' The word signifies the personification of forces of nature, such as eclipses, etc. In later Vedic periods the asuras were regarded as demons that are always in conflict with the devas.

ASURA-MAYA
An Atlantean astronomer/astrologer who authored an ancient text: *Surya-siddhanta*, 'The Power of the Sun.'

ASVINI MUDRA
A technique for opening the sphincter muscle.

ATHARVA VEDA
One of the four ancient sacred scriptures containing formulas for mental and astral purification.

ATMA(N)
The true Self, in contrast with individuality, personality, or body. This is the ever-present, universal Spirit which is free from all conditioning. In the Vedantic philosophy, the Atma is singular and it exists in entities that appear to be separate; it is often called Jiva, or Jivatma. In the Sankhya-Yoga philosophy the technical term is Purusha. In this philosophy there are innumerable Purushas.

AUM (OM)
The sacred symbol which first appears in the Upanishads as a mystical tri-syllable regarded as the basis of all mantras. It is also the root syllable of origination and dissolution. It is also written OM; esoterically it is written AUMM. All that exists is only a development of this eternal syllable. The past, the present and the future are all included in this mantra sound. All that exists beyond the three forms of time is

also implied in this syllable.

It is often used as a mantra as well as a yantra (in the Sanskrit script). This mantra, when chanted properly by a person who has undergone spiritual purification, induces great harmony known as 'Shanti.' This mantra is made up of three sounds: A, U, and M. The two vowels, A and U, blend to produce an O sound; the M is sounded without parting the lips.

This mantra sounds like the word *home* without the H sound, but the sound is prolonged to induce a meditative state. The A mantric sound is made at the back of the mouth, whereas the M sound is made at the front of the mouth with the lips; the U sound is a glide sound between them. This mantra covers the whole range of possible utterances, and thus the word AUM or OM symbolizes all knowledge expressible. AUM also symbolizes the three devas or high celestial beings: Lord Brahma, Lord Vishnu and Lord Shiva, respectively.

AUM TAT SAT AUM (OM TAT SAT OM)
A watchword 'mantra' which symbolizes the Reality.

AVA-STHAS
Refers to the three stages of consciousness that all earthlings have experienced. These are:

The waking state (jagrat), in which one is aware of the external world and its objects, and the so-called objective existence.

The dreaming state (swapna), in which one is aware of the internal world and its objects, and the so-called subjective existence.

The deep sleep state, or the dreamless state (sushupti), in which there is neither an objective nor a subjective existence, only blissful rest.

There is a fourth state which few earthling have experienced. It is called 'turiya.' The key difference between the third and the fourth states is that in the third the sleeping person is still apart from his own True Self. In the fourth stage the individual is no longer apart from, but a part of his True Self.

AVATARA
Avatara literally means 'descender or incarnation from above.' It is the idea that Lord Vishnu has many incarnations, of which ten are most significant. The cycle repeats itself in every age. At the present time, Lord Vishnu has manifested as the ninth avatara, Lord Buddha. The tenth and final avatara of this age will be Lord Kalki. Then the cycle begins again. Each avatara is concerned with an epoch-mak-

ing change in the world. An avatara appears when the world-cycle is at its low point, and needs additional spiritual energy to re-lift the cyclic course of human history.

AVIDYA
Forgetfulness or ignorance which causes error. The basic forgetfulness regards your being Spirit, not matter; your being a part of Reality, not apart from that Reality. Secondarily, it is mistaking that which is temporal as the eternal. Thirdly, it is confusing the Self with the not-self.

AVYAKTAM
Means the unmanifested. *Vyakta* means 'that which is manifested.' Life is spread out before us, and thus we can see it. Because we can only see a small part of life at any given time, we are limited. This limitation is the blessing. By this very limitation we are learning to live. By this very limitation of knowing, we are gaining the strength to know. By this very limitation of consciousness, we are gaining the strength to become more conscious. These various limitations force us to exercise our awareness and thus unfold. This is the secret of living. This is the goal and the reason that life is as it is.

BADDHA-PADMA
The locked-lotus pose.

BAHYA-ABHYAN-TARA KUMBHAKA
Full chalice/empty chalice breath hold.

BANDHA
Muscular contractions to gain control over the life-force in the physical body.

BASTI
Colon cleansing.

BAUDHIKA AHIMSA
Intellectual non-violence.

B.C.E.
Means 'before the common era.'

BENARES
See *Varanasi*.

BHAGAVAD GITA
One of the great scriptures of the world. It is a small book of 18 short chapters. The *Gita* is taken from a much larger work. It is the 11th chapter of the *Mahabharata*, one of the great epics of India. The other epic is the *Ramayana*. Each chapter of the *Gita* deals with the development of the whole person: the physical, the mental, the emotional, the ethical, and the spiritual.

BHAGAVAT
The Lord.

BHAKTA
A devotee practicing bhakti.

BHAKTI
Means 'love or devotion.' It is one of the paths to commune with God.

However, most often the bhakti sect feeds emotions, and thus the experiences, if any, are highly charged emotional experiences. One needs to move from love (bhakti) to 'higher love' (para-bhakti). It is through para-bhakti that the devotee realizes God is not impersonal, but supra-personal. The other path is the path of knowledge (jnana).

BHARVA CHAKRA
The wheel of existence which shows that life is cyclical.

BHASTRIKA
The bellows breath.

BHAVA
Refers to the three outward, manifested states of personality.
The first is *The Bound* (pashu-bhava). The personality is selfish and materialistic. It has little effectiveness in thought, speech, or action.
The second is *The Strong* (vira-bhava). The personality is effective in doing things selfishly or unselfishly.
The third is *The Sacred* (sattwa-bhava). The personality is unselfish in all actions.

These three types of personalities relate to the three qualities (gunas).

BHRAMARI
The bee breath.

BHRIGU
A sage, the son of Brahma.

BHRINGA
The black bee pose

BHRUMADHYA DRISHTI
The frontal gaze technique for concentrating.

BHUJANGA-SAN or BHUJANA
The cobra pose.

BIJA MANTRA
The sounds connected with the tattvas or material principles of each chakra. When the mantric bija sound is chanted, it will psychically be followed by an after-sound which is a nasal M. Thus the Saturn

chakra's bija mantra LA, with its after-sound, becomes LAM. The Jupiter chakra's bija mantra VA, with its after-sound, becomes VAM. The Martian chakra's bija mantra RA, with its after-sound, becomes RAM. The Venus chakra's bija mantra YA, with its after-sound, becomes YAM. The Mercury chakra's bija mantra HA, with its after-sound, becomes HAM.

BINDU
Means a point or dot. It has three major meanings. In mantra, there is often a nasal sound. This is indicated by a dot on top of one of the nasal sounds, generally 'M.'

The second meaning is the source point of creation, most often utilized or symbolized by mantra or yoga-siddhi.

The third meaning of the word is 'semen.'

BRAHMA (SRI)
The principle of creation; the god of creation, one of the Hindu Trinity (Brahma, Vishnu, and Shiva). Brahma, the god of creation, is not to be confused with Brahman, the Reality. Nor is Brahma to be confused with brahmin, the highest group in the caste system. Brahma is the principle of creation, and is represented as sitting on a fully blossomed lotus flower which rises on a long stalk from the navel of the great deity from whom Brahma has his source.

BRAHMACHARYA
The fourth of the abstinences. It means the avoidance of sexual actions, or sexual excitement. The theory is that the energy saved is accessible for higher creative purposes.

BRAHMA-DATUN KRIYA
A type of stomach cleansing using a long string.

BRAHMAN
The ultimate substratum of the universe. Brahman has two manifestations: Saguna Brahman with manifestations, and Nirguna Brahman, the Existent One, which has no qualities. It is said that the immensity of this divine Reality is beyond the comprehension of man, not because of man's limited comprehension, but because only the most minute fragment is ever manifest. Brahman is the essence of all things. Man can approach Brahman only through His minor manifestations, called the deities. Brahman is an indivisible unity and hence is called Purnam: the full and complete.

BRAHMANA TEXTS
Branches of the Vedas consisting of treatises relating to prayer and sacrificial ceremony.

BRAHMA-NADI
Brahma-nadi means 'the river of God.' It is also known as the *sushumna*. It is the most important astral river or nadi situated in the very center of your astral body. This nadi leads to the Brahma-randhra or the Doorway to God. The sushumna is considered to be the divine channel or nadi in the astral body which goes straight up the interior of the spine into the interior of the head, starting from the Saturn chakra. Inside the sushumna is an even finer channel which is called *vajrina-nadi*, and inside this is still a finer channel called *chitrini*. It is this chitrini that the Kriya or the Kundalini ascends from the Saturn chakra to the Door of God. On the left side of the sushumna is the ida, and on the right side is the pingala. These three coil upward and unite at the ajna chakra. The three are symbolized by the caduceus and also all other trinities.

BRAHMA-RANDRHA
The Doorway of God.

BRAHMA-SUTRAS, THE
A text written by the sage, Veda Vyasa, which expounds on the nature of the Reality. The concepts or key teachings are from the *Upanishads*.

BRAHMA-VIDYA
The knowledge of the Reality (Brahman). Also called Brahma-jnana.

BRAHMIN
Refers to a person known as a *brahmana*. He is a man of the highest caste. However, according to the Upanishads, a person should not be defined a brahmin because of social status (as in most of India), but should be defined as a person who is directly aware that he is Spirit (Atma).

BRUMADHYA DRISHTI
A technique of gazing at the Sun center while the eyelids are half opened.

BUDDHI

Means 'comprehension.' The term buddhi denotes the higher mind, or the wisdom component, as contrasted to the lower mind (manas). The buddhi is the subtlest and the deepest feature of the psyche.

Buddhi also means the first derivative of *pre-matter* matter known as prakriti. It is the first most sublime and elementary form of matter. Thus, it gives rise to all other spectrums of 'formed' matter: the so-called material and mental.

CHAKRA(S)
Mass-energy-converters which are also known as wheels, lotuses, or padmas because of their resemblance to the lotus flower. Although there are 72,000 chakras, seven are considered to be the most significant. They are threaded upon the subtle sushumna channel at various levels along the spinal column. They are:

1. The *Saturn chakra* at the base of the spine, called muladhara chakra.
2. The *Jupiter chakra* at the level of the small of the back, also known as swadhisthana chakra.
3. The *Martian chakra* at the level of the navel, called manipuraka chakra.
4. The *Venus chakra* at the level of the heart, known as the anahata chakra.
5. The *Mercury chakra* at the level of the throat, known as the vishuddha chakra.
6. The *Sun chakra* or *single eye* at the root of the nose between the eyebrows called the ajna chakra.
7. The *Moon chakra* known as the chandra chakra. It is at the same level as the Sun chakra. The Sun is at the front of the head, and the Moon at the back.

There is a tendency to relate chakras to the important nerve plexuses. These would be the sacral, prostatic, epigastric, cardiac, pharyngeal and the plexus cavernosus. The padmas or lotuses have petals which indicate the number and types of spiritual energies contained within that chakra. Each petal has one of the 50 letters of the Sanskrit alphabet upon it.

The Saturn chakra has four petals, the Jupiter chakra has six, the Martian chakra has ten, the heart or Venus chakra has twelve, the Mercury chakra has sixteen, and the Sun or ajna chakra has two petals. Over and above this, at the very top of the sushumna, there is a crown chakra called the thousand-petalled lotus. Twenty levels times the fifty lower chakra petals equals the 1,000 petals above.

CHAKRA ASAN
The wheel pose.

CHAMA-GADARA
The bat pose.

CHANDRA (SRI)
The Moon.

CHANDRA BHEDANA
The Moon-piercing breath.

CHANDRA CHAKRA
The Moon chakra. (See *chakra*.)

CHANDRA DHAUTI
A tongue cleansing technique.

CHANDRA NAMASKAR
The salutation to the Moon posture.

CHATUR-MUKHI
The four-phase liberation breath.

CHATUSH-PADA
The lizard pose.

CHELA
A disciple.

CHINMATRA (CHIT-MATRA)
Means pure consciousness and expresses the Transcendental Essence, or the True Self (Atma).

CHIT
Means 'pure consciousness.' It should not be confused with the lower mind, or mind-stuff (chitta). Consciousness is that which is aware of both the body and the mind, and is not to be confused with either. Consciousness is conscious of both the body and the mind, and in Indian psychology, both the body and the mind are not conscious.

CHITTA
The lower mind, or mind-stuff. It is this section of the mind that we must first master. It is in the mind-stuff that all the sensations experienced in a lifetime are stored as information (correct and incorrect), and are available for use when needed.

CHITTA-VRITTI-NIRODHA

The control or stopping of the vacillations of the activity in the lower mind. This is attained by the practice of concentration, meditation, and contemplation.

DAHARA
Refers to the most subtle space within the Venus or heart chakra (anahata), which encompasses the 'linking-point' of the mind/body, and the Transcendental Self.

DAHYA
External pranayama.

DAMA
The control of the body. Or more accurately, the 'becalming' of the ten body organs, five of sense and five of action, so they become and remain quiet when not needed. Dama is one of the six attainments (shat-sampatti) that each student seeks to attain.

DANA
Charity.

DARSHANA
The word means 'to look at,' and in a philosophical sense it refers to the six orthodox schools which are grouped together as they nourish each other. These are: Sankhya-Yoga, Nyaya-Vaisheshika, and Mimansa-Vedanta. The term also refers to the darshan of the Guru. It sees the Guru as having a special blessing. It also refers to a vision state attained by deep inturning.

DATTA-TREYA (SRI)
A hermit; an ascetic; famous in many of the Puranas. He is a symbolic combination of the three devas: Brahma, Vishnu, and Shiva, indicating a movement toward a blending of the three different sects. He is represented either as Brahma, Vishnu and Shiva side by side, or, sometimes as a four-armed Vishnu with the vehicles of Shiva and Brahma. Datta-treya is accompanied by four dogs.

DEHA
Means 'body.' The word *upadi* is also used, but its connotation is more of a *mark* than a body. Therefore, it is that which marks a person's presence; it is that by which a soul is known. The word *sharira* is also used to mean body. An earthling has three bodies:

A dense or gross body (sthula sharira),
A subtle body (sukshma sharira), and
A causal body (karana sharira).

The earthling's marks or expressions are:
His essential state of mind (sanjna),
His qualities (gunas),
His actions (kriyas), and
His status in the world (jati).

In an exoteric sense, his status (jati) materializes from his past-life karma. His actions are done by the dense body. The qualities are contained within his subtle body, and his essential state of mind, or the degree of awakening, is contained in his causal body.

DERGHA-SHVASA-PRASHVASA
Deep breathing.

DEVA(S)/DEVI(S)
A Sanskrit name for celestial or heavenly beings. Deva has been incorrectly translated as *god*. It means a celestial energy. It is the personification of natural forces in the universe, as well as within the human body. Deva indicates a masculine principle; devi indicates a feminine energy. For each deva there is a counter-balancing devi.

Deva comes from the root *div*, meaning 'to shine,' and thus is regarded as the source of all divine energies. The Rig Veda points out that there are 33 devas equally divided among the three lokas or worlds: the earth world, the air world, and the sky world.

Devas are different aspects or facets of the Reality. The Rig Veda states: 'Great is the single Godhead of the devas.' From this arose the Upanishadic doctrine of the one Reality manifesting itself in countless divine forms. Although the Godhead is beyond the spheres of name and form, the Reality can be approached only by means of audible, visible and tangible means.

Each deva is distinguished by his particular attributes, but the chief characteristic of any deva is the capacity to give. Therefore, everything that humans receive, apart from their own efforts, is given by the celestials, or devas. In yogic terms, everything that is received is by the result of one's own karma, and therefore the devas are only the means of the fruition of that karma.

Initially, the only immortal deva was Agni, but in later times immortality was bestowed upon all major Vedic divinities. This occurred when they drank the sacred soma elixir related in the churning of the ocean symbology.

DEVA-DATTA
One of the secondary or minor pranas or vital airs.

DEVA-NAGARI
Divine writing. The characters in which Sanskrit is written.

DHANAN-JAYA
One of the secondary or minor pranas or vital airs.

DHANURASAN
The bow pose.

DHARANA
Concentration. The holding of the mind to one point through effortful use of the mind. Concentration can be looked upon in two ways: narrowing the field of attention, or focusing of the mental powers. Concentration is, doing at will, over a long period of time, what is commonly done spontaneously whenever attention is paid to a thought or object.

DHARMA
This key word has many different meanings, all of which are difficult to translate. It means 'that which sustains and upholds.' It means living a life of high conduct. It means moral duty, religious duty, universal law, universal order, custom, principle, justice, and religion, etc. It means being true to one's own self, often expressed as duty to oneself. It also means duty to one's civilization. It means law, or the proper way of performing ceremony. There are detailed guidelines on how to pray, how to meditate, how to perform devotional subordination (puja), as well as performing sacrificial ceremonies in order to obtain positive, specific results. These laws compose a science for dealing with the forces of the Unseen World. It even includes concern for others as a fundamental extension of oneself. Lord Shiva's bull, Nandi, symbolizes the divine dharma which is firmly established on four feet: Truth, Purity, Compassion, and Charity. All these notions associated with the meaning of dharma are personified in a deva of the same name.

DHARMA-MEGHA
The ninth level of samadhi.

DHAUTI
Means 'cleansing of the physical body.' These techniques are more often used in hatha yoga than in the other yogas. Cleansings are used to purify the physical body, whereas mudras are used to purify the astral body. Both are steps towards the attainment of yogi-siddhi. Some of the physical cleansings can be quite dangerous, and thus should only be practiced after being learned directly from a Guru.

DHRUVA-ASAN
The Sage Dhruva pose.

DHYANA
Meditation. It is meditative examination of the truths heard or read.

DIRGHA-SUKSHMA
The extended forceful breath.

DITARITA-PADA-MASTAKA-STARSHA
The soles-on-head pose.

DRASHTA (DRASHTRI)
A term that Patanjali uses to refer to the Self as the On-Looker, or Witness of the flow of cognitive phenomena. It is this flow of psychomental phenomena that draws the Self away from the Self because it thinks itself to be this psychomental energy. He is, in truth, pure consciousness, and not the content of consciousness.

DRIK
The Seer, the Atma, the Jiva, the Brahman, the Witness. In short, that which sees manifestation.

DRISHYA
Manifestation as contrasted with the See-er of that manifestation. Drishya means 'that which is seen.'

DUMO-FIRE (TUMO-FIRE)
The heat descending over the astral spine. The dumo-fire is released by the Sun and the Mars chakras.

DVAITA
Duality. The first effect of ignorance is to think that we are apart from the rest of life, rather than a part of life.

DVAPARA YUGA
The cycle following the Kali Yuga. It is twice as long and twice as positive as the Kali cycle.

DVESHA
Aversion of an object or an idea.

DVIJA
A 'twice-borne,' i.e., a person invested with the sacred thread.

EKA-CHITTA
Eka means 'one' and *chitta* means 'mind.' Therefore, it means 'of one mind,' i.e., one fixed thought on a concept.

EKA-INDRIYA
One organ detachment. Stage three of sense-withdrawal.

EKA-PADA-PASCHI-MOTTANA
One-leg posterior stretch.

EKA-UTTANA-PADA
The one-leg lift.

ETHER
One of the five primary elements. These are: earth (prithivi), water (jala), fire (agni), air (vayu), and ether (akasha). Ether is sometimes referred to as sky-matter. Air manifests from ether; fire from air; water from fire, and earth manifests from water. From ether down to earth, there is a gradual precipitation or descent into greater density. These five elements are also referred to as great elements or mahabhutas, however, the elements known to us are not great, but are gross and visible.

Gross earth is made up of 50% pure earth and 12-1/2% of each of the other four elements.

Gross water is made up of 50% pure water and 12-1/2% of each of the other four elements.

Fire is composed of 50% pure fire and 12-1/2% of each of the other four elements.

Gross air is composed of 50% pure air and 12-1/2% of each of the other four elements.

Gross ether is composed of 50% pure ether and 12-1/2% of each of the other four elements.

The Sanskrit word for ether is *akasha,* and it is the akashic record or the ethereal space which holds the memory tract of each individual soul, as well as of the universe.

EVA
Verily.

There are no Sanskrit words beginning with the letter 'F.'

GAJA
The elephant pose.

GAJI-KARNI
The dangerous technique of drinking large quantities of water mixed with salt for the purpose of cleansing the physical body.

GAMDHARA
A symbolic, quasi-divine, fabulous half-bird, half-horse; sometimes half-bird, half-man. The Hindus and the Buddhists regard them as benefic beings which confer boons on those with whom they come into contact. Therefore, the yogi who can bring the kriya current up through the gamdhara nadi will receive mystical and spiritual boons.
     On a deeper level, gamdhara is the guardian of the celestial soma. Therefore, the yogi who can move the Kriya current through this nadi will attain soma: the nectar of immortality.

GANDHARVA
A collective group of high astral beings that are generally known as the guardians of the amrita or celestial nectar, which when drunk, releases the spiritual rain cloud productive of fructification of the spiritual efforts.

GANGA (GANGES)
The most sacred river in India; its personification as a goddess, symbolizes purity derived from the primordial waters. Ganga is regarded as a boon sent from heaven. In yoga, the Ganga is the Kriya energy flowing in the sushumna nadi. Therefore, one who bathes in this sacred river attains Enlightenment.

GARUDA
The eagle pose.

GAYATRI MANTRA
The most sacred of all Hindu mantras. In ancient days it was only chanted by Brahmins. It begins: '*Om, bhur, bhuvah, svah.*' The main exoteric meaning of this mantra is, 'We meditate on the Ineffable Effulgence that is the Resplendent Sun. May that Sun direct our Intuition and Insight.' The key concept is that we are not to project our thoughts to these higher states, but rather are those states from which we will receive our blessings.
   Gayatri also refers to the meter in which this mantra is composed.

GHERAND
A sage who compiled or composed the *Samhitas*.

GNANA MUDRA (JNANA)
A mudra formed by joining the index finger to the middle of the thumb. It is a symbol of wisdom.

GOMUKHA
The cow pose.

GORAKSHA
An ancient yogic sage.

GORAKSHA ASAN
The ankle-knee pose.

GORAKSHA PADDHATI
A text written by the Sage Goraksha.

GRANTHI
Means 'knot.' There are three knots in the astral spine. One at the base of the spine in the Saturn chakra. One at the heart level in the Venus chakra, and another at the eye-brow level in the solar chakra. After the Kriya-kundalini is awakened, it has to break through these three knots as it ascends the astral spine. The knot in the Saturn chakra is called the Knot of Brahma. The knot in the Venus chakra is called the Knot of Vishnu. The knot in the Sun center is called the Knot of Shiva.

GUNA
The three qualities of nature: tamas (darkness, laziness, stability), rajas (emotionality, heat, restlessness), and sattva (light, wisdom, orderli-

ness). Tamas is best related as the quality in nature called static inertia. It is symbolized as darkness. It causes things to remain the same. In man it is symbolized as sluggishness, laziness or apathy. The rajas guna is the quality in nature which causes a thing to continue its movement. In mankind it is emotionality, restlessness, or excitability. The third and highest guna is called sattva. The sattva guna is the quality which causes a thing to establish balance in nature. The three gunas are also perceived as subdivisions of maya; thus the veiling quality is tamasic, the projection is rajastic, and the purpose of it all is sattvic. For liberation to manifest, it is necessary for the yogi to transcend above these three gunas.

GUPTA
The celibate pose.

GURU
Dispeller of darkness; a preceptor who takes on the responsibility of the spiritual unfoldment of another soul.

GURU-DEVA
Divine spiritual teacher.

GURU-PARAM-PARA
The apostolic successors of a spiritual Guru.

HA
(See *bija-mantra.*)

HALASAN
The plough pose.

HAMSA
Swan or goose. Hamsa is the spirit that migrates from body to body just as wild geese migrate from place to place (at the correct season).

HANUMAN
One of the heroes of the epic, the *Ramayana*, who has the form of a monkey, which is the symbol of the mind, among other things.

HANUMAN-ASAN
The monkey pose.

HARI
One of the names of Lord Vishnu, the principle of preservation. The indwelling Lord, and the remover of all ignorance.

HARI-OM
A three-lettered mantra.

HASTA-SHIRAKA
The palm-stand pose.

HASTIJIHVA
One of the secondary nadis.

HATHA YOGA
One of the many forms of yoga. Exoterically it deals more with body postures and breathing patterns symbolized by '*ha*' which relates to the Sun, and '*tha*' which relates to the Moon. Hatha yoga is generally considered a first step to the mastery of the mind. Many people, however, bypass this step and go directly into the practice of raja yoga.

HIRANYA-GARBHA
The Golden Womb. It has many meanings which range from the name of the first teacher, or founder of yoga, to the Lord who upholds heaven and earth. It also means 'the first-born' in an evolutionary series. It also means 'the higher mind,' i.e., mahat or buddhi.

HONG-SAU
Manifestation of prana which is the circulation of the solar energy, 'I am that.'

HORA-SHASTRAS
The sacred texts dealing with 'time,' and the correct time for the manifestation of karma.

HRID-DHAUTI
A tongue-cleansing massage.

HUM
Two mantra sounds blended together: the OM mantra of the Sun center, and HA mantra of the Mercury chakra. Blending these two sounds together properly symbolizes the blending of the microcosmic mind with the Macrocosmic Mind.

ICHCHHA-SHAKTI
The power of the 'will' over thoughts and emotions, but even over events in one's life. In its highest level it has the power to sustain control over things. It is the key power which lies behind all concentration.

IDA
A primary nadi located on the left side of the sushumna in the astral body, and ending in the left nostril at the ajna chakra. In yogic terminology, ida and pingala are the ascending and descending channels of the autonomic nervous system. These two pathways function to open both the subconscious and the superconscious minds of the yogi.

IDA-ARDHAMATSYA-INDRA
The left half-spinal twist.

IDA-BHARAD-VAJA
The left sway pose.

IDA-JATHARA-PARI-VARTANA
The left prone spinal twist

IDA-MATSY-INDRA
The left spinal twist

IDA-PRANAYAMA
Empty chalice.

INDRA (SRI)
King of the devas, the lightning-bolt devas.

INDRIYAS
The ten bodily organs by which one gains 'knowledge' of the world. Five of these are the sense organs (jnana indriyas), such as seeing, touching, etc. The other five are the organs of actions (karma-indriyas), such as speaking, walking, etc. The average earthling spends his whole life living in these ten organs.

ISHTA DEVATA
An individual's personal form which symbolizes the deity of that person. The Ishta Devata is also known as the guide who assists the seeker to attain his final goal: samadhi. As various devotees are at different stages of spiritual unfoldment, they will see the impersonal Reality in different forms. This different form, for each soul, is known as the Ishta Devata.

ISHTA MANTRA
The mantra of your Ishta Devata which produces a feeling most harmonious to your inner soul.

ISHVARA (SRI)
The divine willer or the internal supreme giver. Ishvara implants himself in every living being and is the true inner immortal ruler. The notion that God rules from the outside is repugnant to the principle and aim of yoga, for it would involve restriction of the individual's choice.

ISHVARA PRANI-DHANA
The attentiveness to the inward Reality. One of the three basic daily practices of Kriya Yoga imparted by Sri Patanjali.

JAGRAT
The waking state of consciousness.

JALA-BASTI
Water colon cleansing.

JALA-DHAUTI
Water stomach cleansing.

JALANDHARA-BANDHA
The technique of pressing the chin onto the chest during a breath-hold.

JALA-NETI
Water nasal cleaning.

JANU
The thigh pose.

JAPA
Means the repetition of a mantra or the repetition of an idea. The japa of a mantra can be produced mentally, or spoken softly or loudly. The most common mantra to be used in this way is OM (AUM). When a mantra is softly spoken it is called *mantra*. When spoken a little louder, it is called *pajan*. When it is spoken very loudly, it is called *kirtan*. When negative thoughts are experienced, one should evaluate or determine whether the negative thoughts are soft, harsh or very harsh. One should then consciously produce very positive thoughts into the mind in order to properly neutralize these negative forces. Mantra also builds a habit of thinking more positively and more constructively in everyday life.

JATHARA-PARIVARTANA
The prone-spinal twist.

JATI
Status in life, or one's status in the material universe. It includes family conditions, as well as social-economic status, and also one's immediate environment.

JIVA (JIVA-ATMA)
A monad. A unit of life. A person's True Self beyond the body and mind factors. It is the opposite of lifeless (jada). In Western thought it would relate to the 'psyche.'

JIVA-MUKTI
A soul liberated before physical death, or that state of liberation while still embodied in the physical body. A jiva-mukti is 'conscious' of the Jiva or Atma, which is quite different from merely thinking about the Jiva or Atma.

JNANA
Means knowledge or wisdom. It can stand for either secular or sacred knowledge. It also stands for learning. The Gita points out three types of jnana:

1. Seeing a single thing as the Reality.
2. Seeing the composite nature of things, but not the underlying Reality.
3. Seeing the Reality in all things.

JNANA YOGA (GNANA YOGA)
The yoga based on attaining knowledge.

JNATRI, JNANA, JNEYA
The knower, the known, and the act of knowing. In the highest mystical states the sages say that these three are one, not three. Some sages state that when these three become one, perfect meditation ensues. Other sages say that when perfect meditation ensues, these three become one.

JYOTHI
Spiritual light. The holy flame waved before a person to bless him by reminding him that the true flame is within each soul.

JYOTISA
One of the six supportive studies of the Vedas, referred to as dangas. It denotes the science of esoteric astrology.

KAIVALYA
Liberation in which pure consciousness is not affected by forms and energies. Everything in this universe is conditioned existence. Liberation alone is unconditioned existence.

KAIVALYA KUMBHAKA
The instinctive hold in the breathing pattern, known as the Illumination hold.

KAKA
The crow pose.

KALA
Means 'time.' The flow of energy that is the cause of all projection and redissolvement.

KALI-YUGA
The present age, the age of ignorance and disorder.

KALKI
The tenth avatara or Incarnation of Lord Vishnu who is yet to manifest.

KALPA
A cycle of time, also called a Day of Brahma consisting of 1,000 yugas, or a period of four thousand three hundred and twenty million earth years.

KAMA
Desire or emotions. Memories of pleasure and pain previously experienced in relationship with objects and persons. These kamas, when spontaneous, are an integral part of each person's karmic heritage. As you consciously and automatically remember the pleasures previously experienced, these thoughts link to the pleasant feelings engendered, and thus, in time, become the karmic generating factor. In yoga, desire is not to be crushed out, but to be purified and used selectively.

The two most destructive desires on the Path are emersion in sensory life and egotistical self-satisfaction.

KAMALALAYA
The place of Kamala, the lotus, the name of Laksmi. It is also the name of the tenth Mahavidya, or the lotus girl who appears as pure consciousness of Self, bathed by the calm waters of fulfillment. She is the symbol of the state of reconstituted unity. She rules over the auspicious zodiacal sign Taurus, and thus the nadi that leads to the mansion of consciousness known as Taurus, which on a deeper level is the treasure house of all the stored memories within the dense-body structure of an entity.

KAMA-RUPA
The form that passion or desire takes.

KAPALA-BHATI
Skull-shining.

KAPATA
The pigeon pose.

KARANA
The primal cause

KARANA SHARIRA
The causal body. It is the first and the subtlest of the three bodies which we have.

KARMA (THE LAW OF)
The simple idea that everything is caused, as in the laws in physics and chemistry, except that the law of karma is not terminated by time. The law of karma is not the law of retribution nor the law of punishment. It is a simple law that says each soul confines himself according to his actions of the past. He who gambles builds an energy to gamble; he who loves builds an energy to love; he who studies builds an energy to study. What you have done in the past gives you a proclivity to redo that in this lifetime. This is the action of karma. All things that happen to you are caused by your past actions. What you do today will modify yesterday and recreate tomorrow. There are three types of karma:

1. *Kriya-mana karma*: the karma that you are consciously making in this present lifetime.
2. *Pra-rabdha karma*: the karma that is to manifest in this lifetime.

3. *San-chita karma*: the total tank of karma to be manifested in future lifetimes.

It is important to know that karma created in the physical world must be worked out in the physical world; karma created in the dream world has to be worked out in the dream world; karma created in the astral world has to be worked out in the astral world. However, karma created in the meditational state, neutralizes karma in all worlds and planes.

KARMA-PHALA
The results or 'fruits' of a given action.

KARMA YOGA
The yoga of conscious worldly actions. Karma yoga is unselfish motivational action. Karma yoga is an action based upon the unselfish concept of the welfare of others. Karma yoga is action motivated by Wisdom and Love.

KARNA-DHAUTI
Ear cleansing.

KARNATIDA
The knee-pressing-ear pose.

KEDARA
A famous Shiva lingum in the form of a natural ice mass. It is also a holy place in the interior of Kurukshtra, the battlefield of the heart. It is said that he who bathes in this holy place will obtain all the fruits of good actions. In yoga, it is a place inside the skull.

KHAGA
The bird pose.

KLESHAS
The kleshas are the five sources of human trouble. They are ignorance, ego personality, desire, aversion, and possessiveness. In Kriya Yoga these five are primarily due to *avidya* which can be translated as 'forgetfulness.' We simply do not remember, and therefore, we take on mistaken ideas. These kleshas, at any given time, can be vigorously obstructing, slightly obstructing, or dormant. They are weakened by the practice of Kriya Yoga. In the later stages of Kriya Yoga,

the kleshas are dissolved away by kriya dhyana: kriya meditation. The purpose of Kriya Yoga, according to Patanjali, is to remove this root cause of suffering and to attain samadhi.

KOSHA
Koshas are vessels in which something is stored or contained. Man is described as having five sheaths or koshas. They are:

1. *Anna-maya-kosha*, the sheath composed of food, the dense physical body.
2. *Prana-maya-kosha*, the sheath composed of prana or of life-essence.
3. *Mano-maya-kosha*, the sheath composed of the higher and lower mind. This includes manas, chitta and kama.
4. *Vijnana-maya-kosha*, the sheath composed of knowledge.
5. *Ananda-maya-kosha*, the sheath composed of bliss.

These five sheaths are not to be confused with the three bodies which also compose man:

The causal body (karana-sharira) contains the ananda-maya-kosha.

The astral or subtle body (sukshma-sharira) contains the vijnana-maya-kosha, the mano-maya-kosha, and the prana-maya-kosha.

The dense or gross body (sthula-sharira) contains the anna-maya-kosha.

KRIKALA (KRIKARA)
One of the secondary or minor vital breaths. These vital breaths or airs work from within the prana-maya-kosha for the mental, physical, and spiritual health of the entity. Krikala is also the pranic energy related to the feeling of hunger and thirst: the need to feed the soul.

KRISHNA (LORD)
The incarnation of Lord Vishnu. He had a blue body. He died in 3,102 B.C.E., which marked the beginning of the Kali Yuga (iron age, dark age, etc.).

KRITA-YUGA
The first of the four ages or periods in the world's existence. Also called the Golden Age where souls are endowed with the four virtues of kindness, devotion, charity, and truth. (See *yuga*.)

KRIYA (KUNDALINI)

The word *kriya* means 'action.' Kriya energy, therefore, is energy brought about by the action of the mind. Kriya Yoga is the science of conscious efforts directed along certain lines of spiritual action. In *Patanjali's Kriya Yoga Sutras*, he lists three mind actions: 1) tapas, 2) svadhyaya, and 3) ishvara-pranidhana.

Tapas comes from a root word which means 'to heat up' or 'to make hot,' as in the kriya fire. In the earlier stages, it refers to purification actions, because it burns up the karmic impurities in the astral body, thus allowing the mind to grasp subtler and more cosmic states of awareness.

Svadhyaya is mental study, which implies not simply reading but studying the material read, as well as meditation upon those thoughts.

Ishvara-pranidhana is a feeling attunement or an attentiveness to the Inner Reality.

Kriya energy is also referred to in Sanskrit as kriya shakti. Kriya shakti means the action of the mind, which is primarily *thought*. Thought is behind all of our actions. All actions manifest from the habits of the thoughts of the past. Kriya shakti is the power of thought over matter. The development of kriya shakti depends upon the power of concentration and meditation of the yogi. Kriya shakti primarily refers to the visualization process of the mind, or concentrated thought-picturing, without thought activity on the secondary level. Kriya shakti on the third level induces materialization of feelings and materialization in the mind.

KRIYA-BAN

A practitioner of Kriya Yoga.

KRIYA-JYOTHI(S)

Disciples and followers of Goswami Kriyananda's philosophy.

KRIYA-MANA-KARMA

The karma that is being created now, in this very lifetime.

KRIYA-SHAKTI

The power of the mind or thought. Kriya-shakti is the power of thought over matter far beyond the normal patterns or power of the average man or woman. When kriya-shakti is used, the results appear to the average person as marvels or miracles. Kriya-shakti depends upon the power of the mind to focus in deep concentration.

KRIYA YOGA
The yoga of efforts directed along certain lines of spiritual action. Kriya Yoga is the only yoga mentioned by Patanjali in his *Yoga Sutras*. Kriya Yoga is composed of three basic building blocks: 1) tapas, 2) svadhyaya, and 3) ishvara-pranidhana.

Tapas is one of the standard observances to be carried out daily by the yogi. The word comes from a root which means to heat up the Kriya fire which releases the Kundalini, bringing about Enlightenment. Tapas has a preliminary purifying action or Kriya, because the heat in the earlier stages burns up the impurities in the astral body that clog the nadis. Once the impurities in the nadis are burned up, the Kriya energy can be released and can flow to and through the various chakras, producing samadhi and enlightenment. The word tapas is often translated 'austerity,' but should never be confused with morti-fication. Patanjali points out in *Yoga Sutras 2,43:* 'From tapas comes the diminishing of the impurities and thus the perfection of the senses.'

Svadhyaya comes from two words: *Sva* meaning 'self,' and *adhyaya* meaning 'to study.' Therefore, it is the studying or the under-standing of one's self. Some teachers interpret this to mean the study-ing of one's own scripture so that one might come to an understand-ing of the true nature of one's own self. In Kriya Yoga, this self-study is best translated as the awareness of the Atma, the High Self.

The final stage is referred to as *Ishvara pranidhana* or the atten-tiveness to Ishvara, the indwelling God. This has a number of steps:

1. The attunement to the bliss that is divinity, and to see this reflected in all things.
2. The searching and finding of God's benefic, divine purpose in all things.
3. The daily attunement or attentiveness of full devotion; right feel-ing with regard to all events, internal or external.

The proper use of these three pillars along with mantra and pranayama releases kriya shakti or the divine energy of the mind-force. The kriya shakti released is primarily directed at the five sources of our igno-rance.

KRIYA YOGA SUTRAS
The four books on Kriya Yoga written by the sage Patanjali.

KSHATRIYA
The warrior class. One of the four classes or castes of people.

KSHETRA
Means the field of manifested consciousness, as well as all the objects in that field. This term is contrasted with the 'Knower of the Field' (kshet-rajna).

KUHU
The name of one of the four daughters of Angiras and Shraddha. It is a personification of the first day of the waxing Moon.
The Kuhu nadi is a secondary nadi used by the yogi to produce an abundance of spiritual wealth. The greatest wealth that any person can have is the recovery of his memory tract.

KUKKUTASAN
The cock pose.

KUMBHAKA
In pranayama, that state in which the breath and the vital air are restrained from flowing either inward or outward. In a more advanced stage, the prana is not allowed to either ascend or descend in the nadis, but is centered in a given chakra—usually the ajna chakra.

KUNDALINI
The coiled power of the central nervous system, in the sushumna, which lies latent in the Saturn chakra at the base of the spine. When Kriya or Kundalini is completely awakened, the chakras give progressive enlightenment to the yogi.
Kundalini is a force described as lying like a serpent in three coils in the cavity in the Saturn chakra at the base of the spine. She lies there with her head blocking the super-fine channel inside the sushumna, called chitrini. This channel goes straight up the spine. In the practice of kriya yoga, laya yoga, or kundalini yoga, she is awakened, ascends this channel, and acts upon the seven chakras which are threaded on this channel. As each chakra is vitalized, it is altered, bringing about 'deep, spiritual effects upon your consciousness. As the kundalini leaves the seven lower chakras, she enters into the thousand-petalled lotus at the very top of the head, producing cosmic consciousness. These three systems of yoga place the key emphasis upon awakening and directing of this latent force in the physical body. Many of the texts dealing with these procedures are referred to as Tantras. These Indian yoga concepts are the foundation of Tibetan Lamaism.

KUNJAR KRIYA
The technique of drinking large quantities of water mixed with salt, and then regurgitating it; used for cleansing the stomach.

KURMA
Kurma means 'tortoise' and is associated with early cosmogonic theories which liken the cosmos to an egg. The tortoise is used to support Mt. Mandara, which was the stick the devas and the asuras used to churn the ocean. The tortoise represents the resting place of the universe. Astral constellations and astral countries are arranged around it in nine divisions. The tortoise always faces east.

Kurma is also one of the minor or secondary pranas. If the yogi can bring the Kriya current up through this secondary nadi, he sees the source of all things.

KURU-KSHTRA
The field of the heart. The Gita begins, 'Kuru-kshtra, Dharma-kshtra.' It means esoterically, 'On the battlefield of my heart's desires, as opposed to the field of my duty, what am I to do?'

LA
(See *bija mantra*.)

LAKSMI
The goddess of learning.

LAPA
The creeper pose.

LATA CHAKRA
A chakra located at the front of the forehead which relates to the pituitary gland.

LAYA YOGA
A yoga stressing the awakening and the directing of latent forces in the Saturn chakra at the base of the spine. It is the same as kriya yoga or kundalini yoga, however, laya yoga more extensively works with ceremonies and images of Indian gods and goddesses. These powers have their own particular function in the macrocosm, and can be called upon to manifest in the microcosm.

LINGA SHARIRA
Same as the astral or subtle body. Also called *sukshma sharira*.

LOKA(S)
The regions or levels of existence of living beings in any given world. The physical loka is called bhur-loka. The next loka is not visible to our physical senses and is known as the subtle world or bhuvar-loka. The highest of the three regions is swar-loka. The swar-loka is often associated with what Westerners call the heavenly worlds. These worlds also have subdivisions, and thus the word 'loka' can also mean the subdivisions of existence within a world.

LOKA-PALA(S)
The guardians of the regions and also of the four cardinal and intermediate points of the compass. It was in Puranic times that their symbology was fully developed. Six loka-palas are mentioned, each with its own overlord. The most critical is Agni, ruler of the East, and its defender, the Kali-naga.

❋❋❋

MAHA-ATMA (MAHATMA)
A title given to earthlings that are believed to be highly developed, spiritually.

MAHABHARATA
The longest epic poem in world literature. One of the two great epic poems from India. The *Gita* is extracted from it. It deals with duty and keeping one's vows. The other epic poem is the *Ramayama*.

MAHABHUTAS
The five material states of matter or 'elements.'

MAHA-VIRA
The Lord's name in Jainism.

MAHAVIRA ASAN
Sri Mahavira pose.

MAHESHVARA (SRI)
Means 'the great Lord: Lord Shiva, the possessor of great spiritual power.' Within Maheshvara are coordinated the three energies from which knowledge arises: understanding (jnana), willing (iccha) and action (kriya). In Kashmirian Shaivism, the concept of Maheshvara means that the world's mind, as will, is related to the process of nature. The world is not a finished product, but is the very movement of nature, reflecting the working of the universal mind.

MAI-STAHIKI-BRAHMACHARYA
Total celibacy.

MAKA
A yoga push-up.

MANA MAYA KOSHA
The mind sheath. (See *kosha*.)

MANAS
The instrument of action in the mind. It is this instrument of action that produces and modifies objective things.

MANAS CHAKRA
A small chakra located between the Martian chakra and the heart chakra.

MANDARA
A mythical white mountain supported by Lord Vishnu in his tortoise incarnation. Mt. Mandara was used by the devas and the asuras to churn the ocean of milk, to gain the essential objects necessary for survival. This ocean represents the unmanifested cosmos, which contains potentially everything necessary to form a new universe. Sri Kubera, the deva of spiritual riches, the Yaksa, Manibhadra and others reside here.

MANDUKA
The frog pose.

MANIPURA
The Venus or heart chakra. (See *chakra*.)

MANO-MAYA KOSHA
The mind sheath. (See *kosha*.)

MANTRA
The word means 'thought form.' Mantra is an instrument of thought. Mantras are sacred formulas or mystical verses that contain within them primary vibratory forces that create mystical states of consciousness.
   Some mystics say that these mystical states of consciousness can manifest in the external world. All sounds made by earthlings carry a mental influence which exerts itself over matter, whether or not the earthling perceives it or not.

MANTRA-KARA
A person having the wisdom to put together sounds to produce states of consciousness or events is known as a 'mantra-maker' (*mantra-kara*).

MANU
The Hindu law-giver.

MANVANTARA
The life or period of a Manu. There are fourteen Manus. Each Manu is

a ruler who controls his own given age or period. Each period consists of 4,320,000 solar years, which is equivalent to 12,000 divine years, or 1/14th of a Day and Night of Brahma. Fourteen such periods constitute an age or a kalpa. Each manvantara has its own Manu, its own Indra (see Marut), and its own rishis.

MARGA
The spiritual path upon which one walks to reach Enlightenment.

MARUT(S)
The storm gods, armed with lightning and thunderbolts. They are the allies of Lord Indra, king of the devas, also known as the lightning-bolt devas. During a battle, Lord Indra made a charm which confused his enemies and the Maruts slew them. The Maruts are often asked to cause darkness to prevent the enemy from seeing each other.

The Maruts are linked with Deva Agni, the fire Lord, and with Deva Vayu, the air Lord. The Maruts are said to roar like lions and have teeth of iron, which also associates them with Nirasimha.

In the Vishnu and the Brahmanda Puranas, there are seven groups of seven, each seven dwelling in one of the seven spheres: the earth, the Sun, the Moon, the stars, the planets, the pole star, and the constellation of Ursa Major. In early Vedic times the Maruts were the first air or atmospheric deities. Their name comes from *ma-rutah*, the measure of sound.

MATHA
A monastery or ashram where people go to learn and practice yoga undisturbed by the outside world. Some enter for life, whereas others enter for a year or so.

MATSYA
The fish pose.

MATSY-INDRA
The spinal-twist pose.

MAUNA
The abstaining from speaking, i.e., the vow of silence. This vow can be anywhere from a few minutes to the total life.

MAURI
The peahen pose.

MAYA

Often inaccurately translated as 'illusion.' The doctrine of maya is that everything experienced in this manifest universe is a projection of the mind, either from the mind of the individual or from the mind of the Cosmic Being. Thus what we see in the physical universe veils something which exists in the divine world but is not perceived in the physical world.

An adjective often used with maya is the word 'indescribable.' It simply means that what we see cannot properly be described as either real or unreal. Metaphysically, any object can only be known through and with the mind that is perceiving the object, and thus the mind, in a sense, interferes with the true seeing.

There are four meanings to the word maya:

1. The power which has produced this universe.
2. That which is composed of the three gunas.
3. That which has no beginning.
4. The power of the divine will.

MAYA-KOSHA

A temporal sheath. (See *kosha.*)

MAYURASAN

The peacock pose.

MERU-DANDA

This is the astral spinal column. In ancient symbolism everything of the universe was produced from an 'Ocean of Milk' in which Mt. Meru stood. The *devas* and the *asuras* took the Great Serpent of Eternity (Time), Ananta, wrapped it around Mt. Meru and pulled on either end. In so doing they turned the mountain and churned the Ocean of Milk from which various magical and meaningful 'things' floated to the top like butter from churned milk.

MERU, MOUNT.

(See *Mount Meru*)

MIMANSA

One of the orthodox schools of philosophy dealing with the principles of formal religion.

MOHA
Delusion which brings confusion, foolishness and thus affliction. The Great Delusion is the mistaken notion that one is a limited identity, rather than the Transcendental Self.

MOKSHA
Liberation, which is the final spiritual goal of the mystic.

MOUNT MERU
Also known as Mt. Su-meru. It is the name of the symbolic golden mountain that is a key subject of numerous Puranic symbolisms. It is the central point of the internal universe. Such mountains are the meeting place or the abode of the devas.

It is from this golden summit that the celestial Ganges falls before dividing into four terrestrial streams moving out to the four points of the compass. The heavenly spheres of Lord Krishna and Lord Vishnu are located on Mt. Meru.

In symbolic terms, Mt. Meru is 756,000 miles tall, and it runs below the surface of the earth to 144,000 miles. The diameter at the summit is 288,000 miles and its base is 144,000 miles. Hence, its shape gives the metaphor of the lotus of the earth.

Brahma's square city of gold is situated on Mt. Meru's summit. On the outskirts of the golden city are the eight holy cities of the eight loka-palas. Beneath this mountain there are seven nether worlds, and in the very lowest of these resides the giant serpent, Vasuki, which is supporting Mt. Meru and all the worlds.

MUDRA
This refers to hand gestures, or more accurately, gestures made with the fingers that are used during certain types of rituals and/or meditations. Many different yoga texts list from 10 to 37 different mudras. The main purpose of a mudra is to 'gather' energy in a given chakra so as to obtain metaphysical visional states and/or psychic powers (yoga siddhis).

MULA-BANDHA
The contraction of the anal sphincter muscles.

MULA-DHARA CHAKRA
The Saturn chakra at the base of the spine. (See *chakra*.)

MUNI
A person who has taken the vow of silence (mauna). However, today it is often used as a term for a yoga philosopher.

MURCCHA
The mind-quieting breath.

NADA
Means 'sound,' but more accurately, a particular type of sound. This is best stated as 'innerward sound' or astral sounds. Historically, there are several astral sounds such as a bee hum, bell, lute, flute, etc. Each sound is at a subtler level. The yogi uses these sounds as mental steps to ascend to the Soundless Sound. The term *nada* also refers to the extension of a mantra sound when chanting.

NADA YOGA
The yoga using sound for the unifying factor.

NADHI
The navel pose.

NADI(S)
Nadi means 'river.' It is the name for the channels in the astral or subtle body through which Kriya and/or prana energy flows.

NADI SOGHANA
The purification of the astral channels.

NADI SUDDHI
The purification of the astral channels.

NAGA
In Hindu symbology, naga is a general term for both snakes and elephants. It is, also, one of the ten vital breaths.

NAMA-RUPA
Means 'name and form,' referring to the character of anything that comes into a state of manifestation. 'Form' refers to the objective existence of an object, whereas 'name' refers to the subjective side of the object. Therefore the term *nama-rupa* refers to the 'reality' of the manifested object as it moves through Time and Space.

NASAGRA-DRISHTI
The technique of gazing at the tip of the nose.

NAULI
An abdominal chakra cleansing technique.

NETI
A nasal cleansing technique.

NIDI-DHYASANA
Profound meditation. It is practiced only after practicing: the reading of sacred text, and thinking about the thoughts in the text.

NIDRA
An idea obtained during the sleep state. For the average person these are 'dream fragments.' For the disciple these can be deep, profound concepts, ideas, ideals, and feelings.

NIRA-SIMHA (NRI-SIMHA)
The lion-headed incarnation of Lord Vishnu in which the lower part of the entity was a man and the upper part of the body was a lion. Nirasimha, or the lion-headed one, is a symbolism for the yogi's mane and a storage place of pranic energy in the ajna chakra. Nirasimha is one of the key symbolisms of Kriya Yoga.

NIRODHA
The control of the ideas in the mind-stuff (chitta). In Patanjali's yoga there are four levels of controlling or restricting the mind-stuff:

1. Restriction of the fluctuations of the mind (vritti-nirodha).
2. Restriction of 'presented ideas' by means of samadhi.
3. Restriction of subliminal, subconscious forces (samskara-nirodha) by means of higher states of samadhi.
4. Total restriction by means of the highest state of samadhi.

NIR-VICHARA SAMADHI
The fourth level of samadhi.

NIR-VITARKA SAMADHI
The second level of samadhi.

NIYAMA
The five observances which are composed of: 1) the cleanliness of body and mind, 2) contentment, 3) study of the Self, 4) Yoga asceticism, and 5) attentiveness to the indwelling Reality. These five practices make it possible for a person to enter into deep contemplation (samadhi).

NYAYA
One of the orthodox schools of philosophy dealing with principles of logic.

OM
(See AUM.) The mantra sound of AUM reminds one that any action taken should be for the betterment of the universe and all sentient beings therein.

OM MANI PADME HUM
A sacred mantra meaning on the exoteric level: 'The Jewel is in the Lotus.'

OM MUDRA
A mudra formed by bringing the tips of the thumb and the index fingers together.

OM NAMA SHIVAYA
This mantra contains the secret of any being which has five senses.

OM NAMO BHAGAVATE VASU DEVAYA
The twelve-lettered mantra.

OM NAMO NARAYANAYA
The eight-lettered mantra.

OM SAHITA RECHAKA
The chanting of OM with exhalation breath.

OM SRI RAM, JAI RAM, JAI, JAI RAM.
This mantra repeated three times gives the 24-lettered mantra.

OM TAT SAT OM
(See AUM TAT SAT AUM.) This mantra is often used at the beginning of an undertaking. TAT (That) refers to the Reality, and reminds the yogi that he is to reject any negative or unworthy action. SAT (Being) reminds him to act with goodness.

PADA-PRASARAN-KACHCHAPA
The tortoise pose.

PADMA
The lotus pose.

PADMA-SHIRA
The lotus headstand pose.

PAJAN
Clear, strong chanting.

PANDAVAS
The five sons of Pandu who fought against the Blind King in the epic of the Maha-bharata.

PARA
Means 'that which is beyond manifested states.'

PARA-BRAHMAN
(See *Alinga.*)

PARAMA-HAMSA
A title given to highly developed Gurus. It means the most perfect gander.

PARAM-ATMA
The Supreme Atma. Because people often use the word *Atma* to mean the lower self and also the higher self, but not the True Self, Param-atma is used to express this True Self.

PARA-SHIVA
(*See Alinga.*)

PARA-VISHNU
(*See Alinga.*)

PARBATA
The mountain pose.

PAR-SHVOTTANA
The head-to-knee side stretch.

PASCHIMATA
The posterior stretch, or forward bend.

PASHUPATI (SRI)
One of the many titles of Lord Shiva; Lord Shiva as the divine herds-man, the great soul who gathers the divine cows (human beings), who are upon the spiritual path.

PATANJALI, SRI
The author of *The Yoga Sutras*. He lived about 200 years before the common era. He is neither the originator nor the original formulator of these Sutras. The text is an extraordinary re-working of a very ancient text. This text has four divisions or chapters: Contemplation, The Practice of Yoga, Yoga-siddhi, and Liberation.

PAVANA-BASTI
Air colon cleansing.

PAVANA MAKTI
A gas relieving technique.

PAYASVINI (PAYASNI)
A holy river. Those who bathe in this river will benefit equal to the amount of a person who gives 1,000 cows to a religious order. It is also one of the secondary nadis.

PINGALA (NADI)
The nadi to the right of the sushumna. This nadi coils around the sushumna and enters the right nostril at the ajna chakra.

PINGALA-ARDHA-MATSYA-INDRA
Right half-spinal twist.

PINGALA-BHARAD-VAJA
Right sway.

PINGALA-JATHARA-PARIVARTANA
Right prone-spinal twist.

PINGALA-MATSY-INDRA
Right spinal twist.

PINGALA PRANAYAMA
Full chalice.

PLAVANI
The floating breath.

POOR DOTTANA
The back bending pose.

PRABIBHA
Intuition or insight.

PRACHHAR-DANA
The forceful exhalation and breath hold.

PRAJAPATI
The Lord of creation. This word comes from *praja* meaning 'propagation,' and *pati* meaning 'Lord.' A Vedic concept symbolizing the personified forces of nature as a single creative force. Prajapati was later merged into the concept of Lord Brahma.

The Puranas point out that Prajapati formed living creatures out of his own sacrificial offerings to the devas, and when these living creatures were destroyed by the Maruts (the storm devas), they were recreated by Prajapati. The Artha Veda identifies Prajapati's creative energy with prana or the vital breath.

In Vedic tradition there are 33 devas, but Prajapati is regarded as the thirty-fourth deva, symbolizing the totality of these 33. The Samhitas point out that Prajapati had 33 daughters, whom he presented to King Soma.

Prajapati is the divine counterpart of the earthly sacrificer. He is also 'time' which leads to death, so that the sacrificer himself might become death, and by that act, overcome death.

According to Sri Manu, the horse is sacred to Prajapati, because He assumed that form when He searched for Lord Agni, who hid in the water of the gods.

Prajapati also means the twelve symbolic great sages, also referred to as maha-rishis: the mind-born sons of Sri Brahma. Prajapatis were also called Brahma-rishis or Brahma-putras, and as such symbolize the instrumentality of the secondary creation. This concept of evolution begins with the notion of the Self-existent One, called Svayambhu: the unknowable and the unfathomable, who divided his own body and became half male and half female. The female half symbolizes the cosmic potency which was produced from the male Viraj. Svayambhu then called into existence the great sages destined to be the lords of all created beings.

PRAJNA
Wisdom containing spiritual understanding. It manifests in the mind of the yogi when he has walked the eight stages of yoga.

PRAKRITI
The word literally means 'the fourth-made.' Prakriti is the primordial material from which matter is made. It is a Shankya-Yoga term used to describe the primordial matter in the physical universe, which divides itself into three types, called gunas. Everything in the universe is made out of prakriti, except the spiritual selves, called purushas.

Prakriti is personified as the active female principle through which the inactive male principle in the universe is manifested. Together, these two constitute nature with its dual function: generation and redissolvement.

PRAKRITI-LAYA
A bodiless state of consciousness. (See *videha*.)

PRA-LAYA
The dissolution of the universe; from the words *pra* meaning 'dissolution,' and *laya*, meaning 'the place of.' It is the dissolving of the world at the end of each kalpa, or at the end of the Day of Brahma. It precedes a new creation or emanation. According to the Vishnu-Purana, there are four kinds of dissolution.

1. Occasional: when the Lord of the world sleeps. (This is called Brahma-pralaya or Brahma's Dissolution.)
2. Elemental: when the world egg reverts to its primary element from which it was derived.
3. Absolute: the absolute non-existence of the world as experienced by the rishi who becomes merged in the super abundant Brahman.
4. Perpetual: the constant disappearance of day and night and of all things that are born.

At the end of 100 years of Sri Brahma's life, the great dissolution takes place called Maha-pralaya, which is ruled over by the goddess Maha-kali (great time). At this time all forms dissolve into the indescribable primordial prakriti from which a new universe emanates.

PRAMANA
The ideas (vrittis) in the mind supported by perception, inference, or testimony, and therefore regarded as correct (for all practical purposes).

PRANA
The life-force or cosmic energy which divides itself into ten vital sub-forces, also called pranas, vital airs, or vital breaths. Of the vital breaths, Prana remains supreme forever and is described as existing in the heart chakra of the ajna chakra. It is sometimes perceived as yellow or coral in color.

PRANA-APANA SAMYKTA
The balancing ascending-descending breath.

PRANA-MAYA KOSHA
(See *kosha*.)

PRANA-YAMA
The control or the correct regulation of the breath. Breath control is composed of four stages: inflow, hold, outflow, and hold. The inflow hold is known as the *full chalice*, whereas the outflow hold is known as the *empty chalice*. These four components are to be regulated according to time, place and number. The number refers to the relationship of the breathing pattern: one count of inbreath, to four counts of hold, to two counts of outbreath.

PRAPTA
That which manifests in a person's life, and which is not the result of his immediate efforts.

PRARAB-DHA
That karma which has 'ripened' and is active in a person's life. Some yogis state that this karma cannot be averted as it is already active. Other yogis say that it can be softened (by attitude, etc.).

PRATI-LOMA
Opposite nadi breath.

PRATYA-HARA
Sense withdrawal, or withdrawal of the senses. It is well-known that when one is deeply engaged in something interesting, loud noises, etc, are not heard. Sense withdrawal is a conscious, deliberate attempt to withdraw from the activity of the external world, so as to gain entrance into the inner world.

PRATYA-KSHA
Direct perception. The state of being able to obtain or use direct perception is a vital essental in order to progress on the spiritual path, as books and words are too limited.

PREM
Unselfish love.

PRITHVI MUDRA
The earth gesture.

PURAKA
Literally means 'filling up.' Puraka is the process of inbreathing in any pranayama.

PURANA(S)
Purana means 'old.' It is a collection of tales from ancient times. Around 500 B.C.E. when Buddhism sprang forth in India, the Buddhistic teachings threatened the Hindu philosophy which was highly technical and philosophical. As a counter-movement, to convey the Vedic teachings to the unlettered, the Puranas were gathered and circulated among the non-Brahmins, including women. The two dynamic forces within the Puranas are Lord Shiva and Lord Vishnu, which represent the two primary schools of Hindu theological thought.
    The Puranas expound five things:

1. The creation of the world.
2. The dissolving and recreation of the world.
3. The geneologies of the devas.
4. The reigns and periods of Manu.
5. The history of the solar/lunar royal dynasties.

With the development of the Puranic school of thought there was a heavy diminishing of interest in Lord Brahma, the creator. Today, only one or two Brahma temples exist in all of India.

There are two groups of Puranic literature: the primary Puranas called Maha Puranas, and the secondary Puranas called Upa Puranas. Each group consists of 18 works. Two of the most important Maha Puranas are the Agni Purana and the Vishnu Purana. The two most important Upa Puranas are Narasimha Purana and Aditya Purana.

PURUSHA
The word means 'Spirit' or 'pure consciousness,' and refers to the real person. Patanjali refers to Purusha as the Onlooker or the Self-aware One. Some yogis call the Purusha, the Self-Existent One.

PURUSHA KHYATI SAMADHI
The seventh level of samadhi. This level is also referred to as: Viveka-khyati, Vivekaja-jnana, or Taraka-jnana.

PUSHA
One of the 14 major nadis.

PUSHAN (SRI)
A nadi of the Sun.

There are no Sanskrit words beginning with the letter 'Q.'

RA
(See *bija-mantra*.)

RAGA
Desire. An emotion of liking and thus of desiring, arising from a memory of pleasure connected with past experiences.

RAJA
The second quality or guna which causes the release of energy. It is often seen as restlessness, or ardent actions.

RAJA YOGA
One of the systems of yoga in which the person declares and affirms himself as the king (raja) of his mental possessions, and thus his astral powers. The aim of this realization of king or master is the attitude of self-dependence, and of not depending on any outside force or being.

RAMA
Lord Rama is the eighth avatara of Lord Vishnu and the hero of the *Ramayana*.

RAMAYANA
One of the two epics of ancient India. It is the story of Lord Rama and his overcoming the negative forces of love and life. The other epic is the *Mahabharata*.

RASHA
Dance. It refers to a mystery dance performed by Guru and disciples. It was also performed by Lord Krishna and the shepardesses.

RECHAKA
Means 'emptying.' It is the outbreathing process in any pranayama technique.

RIG VEDA
The oldest of the sacred books. They are a repository of symbolic, sacred lore.

RISHI
A sage or seer that is, or was, inspired, leaving behind a legacy of sacred writings.

RUDRA (SRI)
The Vedic Lord of the tempest whose characteristics are thunder and lightning. Sometimes Sri Rudra is directly identified with Lord Agni and Lord Indra. Sri Rudra's key function is to manifest spiritual rain.

RUPA
Form.

SA-BIJA
Means 'with seed.' It refers to those structures of meditation and samadhi which result in a new level of awareness regarding the object of meditation.

SACHCHIDANANDA (SAT-CHIT-ANANDA)
The nature of the Reality, called 'That' (Tat) in yoga.

SADHANA(S)
The yogic practices which are methods for attaining spiritual goals. The highest of these goals is Liberation. There are four key means to Liberation:

1. Willing liberation (mumuk-shutva) from limitations of the worldly life. This is the awakening of spiritual hunger and thirst.
2. Discernment (viveka) between the Atma and the temporary bodies or self-images caused by the thoughts and emotions of the lower mind. It is the discernment of the Self-Existent One from the sevenfold mind/body complex: the four bodily conditions of pain, pleasure, desire, and aversion, and the three mental conditions of thought, feeling and willing.
3. Detachment or dispassion (vairagya), which is an effort not to color events by your emotions caused by negative past habits and present circumstances. This gives clear, unbiased thinking.
4. The six accomplishments (shat-sampatti) toward which the disciple directs his determination and self-discipline:

   a. Control of the mind, producing calmness (*shanti*) by spiritual understanding of the value of all experiences.
   b. Control of the body (*dama*) to produce harmony, rather than impulsive or lethargic actions.
   c. Removal of eagerness (*uparati*); not acting on the basis of mere customs.
   d. Patience (*titiksha*), endurance, and forbearance without anxiety, antagonism or resentment.
   e. Confidence (*shraddha*) in life.
   f. Steadiness of mind; one-pointedness directed toward one goal (*samadhana*).

SAHAS-RARA PADMA

The thousand-petalled lotus. It is not a chakra, but a lotus, and exists at the top of the astral spinal column, in the astral brain. Each petal has one of the 50 letters of the Sanskrit alphabet on it, and these are repeated 20 times. The thousand-petalled lotus pertains to the Paramatma itself. In short, it is the place of the unmanifested Lord Shiva. When the Kundalini enters the padma, and then descends through the chakras, the Kundalini rejuvenates the powers of the chakras which were latent.

SAHITA KUMBHAKA

Full chalice/empty chalice. Holding the breath when the lungs are filled, and holding the breath when the lungs are empty.

SALABHA

The full locust pose.

SAMADHI

Known as contemplation. It is the highest and last stage of yoga. Samadhi cannot be developed by desiring or by will power! It is attained only through tapas and self-discipline. There are two types of samadhi: cognitive samadhi and non-cognitive samadhi. Cognitive samadhi has two sub-forms:

1.   Observation and inquiry,
2.   Reasoning and investigation.

One might say that samadhi is the opposite of going to sleep. It is the state of wakefulness or superconsciousness. It is the perfect union of the Self with the Reality. The prerequisites to the attainment of samadhi are non-violence and contentment. Without these building blocks, all spiritual exercises are doomed to failure.

Although there are many levels and types of samadhi, there are two main divisions:

1.   *Sam-praj-nata samadhi*, in which the yogi has identification with the object of meditation.
2.   *Asam-praj-nata samadhi*, in which the yogi has identification with the Transcendental Self.

Another way of saying this is: in the first type of samadhi the yogi is aware of the content of consciousness. In the second type of samadhi the yogi is only aware of consciousness.

SAMANA
One of the major vayus or vital breaths.

SAMATVA
Means 'equality of the mind.' This state exists when all antagonism and discontentment is no longer alive in the mind.

SAMA VEDA
The fourth and last *Veda*. It centers upon religious chants used by priests during a ritual. These chants are mostly taken from the *Rig Veda*, and modified to suit liturgical conditions.

SAMA-VRITTI
Identical motion breath.

SAMHITA(S)
Means a collection of texts arranged and composed much like, or similar in character to, the *Rig Veda.*

SAM-PRAJNATA SAMADHI
The state of samadhi which has seed. This means that the consciousness is still fixed upon the content of the container.

SAMSARA
The course of human experience and existence through incarnation after incarnation. Egocentric-wise, it implies moving through the same set of thought-patterns, again and again.

SAMSKARA
A samskara is a deep subconscious habit or mood from a past life(s), which acts as an activator of the karma of this lifetime. Samskaras cause a person to act in an automatic fashion.

SAMYAMA
Inquiry into an idea or object by means of blending the methods of concentration, meditation and contemplation ... taken in succession.

SAN-CHITA
That karma which is in storage, awaiting an opportunity to manifest. This type of karma can be softened and even prevented by wise actions and skillful means.

SANKHYA
One of the orthodox schools of philosophy dealing with principles of the classification of the universe. This school of thought was propounded by the sage Kapila. It is closely linked with Yoga philosophy.

SANNYASA
Renunciation, or putting aside possession and worldly activities.

SANNYASI
A soul who has totally renunciated the world. A true sannyasi is a person who renounces the 'fruit' of his actions. In short, he acts without desire for gain (emotionally, or otherwise).

SANTOSHA
Contentment. One of the five observances. In my opinion, this is the most essential psychological attitude to attain if spiritual progress is to be made.

SAPTA VYAHRITA
Mantra regulated breathing.

SARASVATI
Exoterically, it is an ancient river in northwestern India, often erroneously identified with the modern Sarasvati River. Esoterically, it is one of the 14 major nadis, and is personified by Sarasvati, the goddess of learning. This nadi is considered 'the best mother, the best of rivers, the best of devis.' Therefore, the yogi who bathes in the Kriya currents of the Sarasvati is cleansed of all impurities and ignorances.

SAR-GARBHA-SAHITA KUMBHAKA
Mantra with retained breath.

SARVA DVARA BADDHA
Solar bound breath.

SAR-VANGA
Shoulderstand pose.

SASHTAN-GADAN-DAVATA
The spiritual prostration pose.

SAT
The Reality, Truth, Brahman.

SAT-CHIT-ANANDA
(See *Sachchidananda*.)

SATTVA
One of the gunas; that of equanimity. (See *guna*.)

SATYA
Truthfulness.

SAVASANA
The total relaxation pose; also called the corpse pose.

SAVI-CHARA SAMADHI
The third level of samadhi.

SAVI-TARKA SAMADHI
The first level of samadhi.

SAVITUR
(See *Surya*.)

SETU BANDHA
The arch, or the bridge pose.

SHABDA
Sound, which is sevenfold.

SHAKTI
The fundamental forces found in the manifest universe. These shaktis or forces are often symbolized as devis. The three key devis are the feminine attributes of the trimurti: Sri Devi Sarasvati is the wife of Sri Brahma and the patron of all knowledge. Sri Mata Lakshmi is the wife of Lord Vishnu, and the devi of prosperity. Sri Mata Parvati is the wife or consort of Lord Shiva, and is the world mother. In one of the myths, she is described as having playfully placed her hands over Lord Shiva's eyes. Immediately another eye appeared in the middle of his forehead to prevent the whole creation from becoming enveloped in darkness.

The flow of manifest spiritual powers does not stop at these three forces. It permeates all levels of life. The shaktis can manifest even as the subtlest forces, indicated by the 50 letters of the Sanskrit alphabet on the petals of the chakras. Relating to the practice of yoga, there

are four powers or shaktis that arise from the practice of yoga. These
are:

1. The first power has to do with the extension of the perceptive
    faculties and develops into states of clairvoyance, clairaudience,
    clairsentience, psychometry and telepathy. This power is called
    jnana-shakti.
2. The second power has to do with the extension of sound, and is
    used in controlling nature, such as rain-making, etc. It is called
    mantra-shakti.
3. The third power has to do with the extension of will power. It
    gives abnormal control over the body, including the ability to es-
    cape from it, as in the case of bi-location and astral travel. It is
    called ich-chha-shakti.
4. The last power has to do with the extension of visualization, how-
    ever, without any background of thought-activity. It gives one the
    ability to materialize whatever is visualized (without thought-ac-
    tivity). It is called kriya-shakti.

SHAMA
Calming of the mind.

SHANKHINI
One of the 14 major nadis.

SHANTI
Means 'equilibrium' or 'peace.' It is most often repeated three times,
each repetition being softer than the one before. It is preceded by
OM: OM, shanti, shanti, shantih. Exoterically, it means, 'May the physical universe be in equilibrium. May the mental universe be in equilibrium. May the causal universe be in equilibrium.'

SHANTI MUDRA
The mudra formed by placing the middle finger on top of the index
finger, using the right hand.

SHARIRA
Means 'body.' The earthling has three bodies: dense or gross (sthula),
subtle or astral (sukshma), and causal (karana). The sub-divisions
within these bodies are called vessels or sheaths (koshas).

SHARIRIK-AHIMSA
Physical non-violence.

SHAT KRIYAS
The six purification techniques.

SHAT-SAMPATTI
The six (shat) accomplishments that are needed upon the path. The student needs to direct his will power and his self-discipline towards these accomplishments. These are:

1. Control of the mind to the degree that it produces stillness and calmness (shama).
2. Control of the physical body (dama).
3. The acceptance of what life offers (from past-life karma), yet spiritually moving forward to improve life.
4. The development of patience regarding arduous conditions (because of one's own karma).
5. The development of confidence in oneself and life (shraddha).
6. The development of one-pointed concentration which is continually directed towards the person's life goal.

SHAUCHA
Cleanliness of mind and body. The first of the five observances.

SHESHA
The serpent which symbolizes 'Time,' which manifests in repetitious cycles so that what a person could not do in one cycle, can be accomplished in another cycle.

SHIRSHA-SAN
The headstand pose.

SHIVA (SRI)
The Lord of re-dissolvement; the protector and benefactor of yogis. Lord Shiva does not have incarnations but has manifestations. He is depicted with either two or four arms. Taurus is his mount.

SHIVA MUDRA
The technique of closing the nostrils in pranayama.

SHIVA-NATARAJ
The dancing Shiva, doing the 'Dance of Life' (and death).

SHLOKA
Verse.

SHRADDHA
Means 'confidence.' It is not blind faith, but confidence due to mystical experiences and philosophical reflection.

SHRUTI
Means 'what has been heard' from a Guru, seer, or a divine source. Later, it began to have the connotation of 'scripture.' *Shruti* contrasts with *smriti*. *Smriti* means 'what has been remembered.' It is of human origin.

SHUKA
The parrot pose.

SIDDHASAN
The adept's pose, which establishes a disposition for stability.

SIDDHI
Occult powers which the yogi can develop or attain. Historically there are eight siddhis which, according to yoga, should not be sought after. However, as certain persons practice yoga, they spring automatically because of past-life karma. It is said that many people lose the path to samadhi by seeking after these powers, or trying to extend them once they manifest. These siddhis are:

- 1-2: To become very small or very large, at will.
- 3-4: To become very light or very heavy, at will.
- 5-6: To manifest any desire; to obtain anything.
- 7: To control anything.
- 8: Mastery to direct affairs by means of the use of the elements. It should be understood that these siddhis are an esoteric tabulaton of the inner control of one's own states of consciousness.

SIMHA
The lion pose.

SIRSHA
The headstand pose.

SITA
Female principle of the chakras. Also, the wife of Lord Rama.

SITALI
The cooling breath.

SMRITI
That which is remembered. The term is often used to refer to old texts containing memories. (See *shruti.*)

SOMA
Soma means 'the mountain born,' or 'brought from the sky by the eagle (Scorpio),' and thus is considered to be of divine origin. It is called the 'nectar of the gods.' It is the name of an esoteric elixir. Its juice, after being spiritually filtered, induces immortality. It was sometimes mixed with milk, water, butter, or barley. It has nothing to do with any elixiogenic drug.

In later philosophy, soma was related to the Moon or chandra. The mystical symbolism of the soma juice of immortality, or the soma ceremony, is related in the Puranic tales of the churning of the ocean. The process of pressing or the crushing of the soma plant between the stone of Capricorn and the stone of Aquarius in the muladhara chakra is only finalized when the juice flows freely as the result of a divine act rather than as a result of physical effort.

SOMA-DEVA
The deva of Soma, also called the devi of the Moon.

SRI
A title of respect originally meaning 'holy' or 'honored.'

STAMBHA VRITTI
The held motion breath.

STHALA BASTI
The earth colon cleansing.

STHULA SHARIRA
The dense or gross body.

SUKHASAN
The pleasant pose.

SUKSAMA SHVASA PRASHVASA
The gentle and soft exhalating breath.

SUKSHMA SHARIRA
The astral or subtle body.

SUPTA VAJRA
The camel pose.

SUPTA VIRA
The supine hero pose.

SURYA (SRI) OR SAVITUR
The two names most frequently used in the *Rig Veda* to denote the Sun and the solar deva. Surya is derived from the Vedic word *svar* meaning 'to shine.' This Sun is symbolized by wheels, disks, chakras, padmas, and open lotus flowers, denoting its creative function.

Surya is the aditya par excellence of all the other 12 adityas and is referred to individually or collectively. All are associated with light and are generally epithets or aspects of the Sun.

Surya represents death as well as life, and is known to be the intermediary between light and darkness. All creatures in terrestrial spheres must inevitably die, because they are subject to time. Those, however, who ascend to the celestial sphere outside of time, attain immortality. Hence, Savitur is the celestial door to immortality, for the Sun is the center of creation, the point where the manifest and the unmanifest worlds unite.

The Upanishads point out that the splendor of Savitur should be constantly meditated upon, because He is the meditator abiding in the intellect.

SURYA BHEDI or SURYA BHEDANA
A Sun-piercing pranayama.

SURYA CHAKRA
A minor chakra located between the Mars chakra and the Venus chakra.

SURYA NAMASKAR
The salutation to the Sun pose.

SUSHUMNA
The most important astral passageway. The center channel through which Kriya energy flows to produce samadhi or cosmic consciousness. This passageway goes straight up the interior of the spine; it

starts from the Saturn chakra and ends inside the skull. Inside the sushumna is a finer passageway called vajrini-nadi. Inside this is still a finer passageway called chitrini-nadi. It is on chitrini that the chakras exist.

SUSHUMNA DRISHTI
Spinal gazing concentration technique.

SUTRA NETI
String nasal cleansing.

SVADHITHANA
The Jupiter chakra. (See *chakra*.)

SVA-DHYAYA
'*Sva*' means 'one's own,' and *adhyaya* means 'study.' Therefore, *svadhyaya* means 'the study of one's own self.' Later, it came to be interpreted, incorrectly, as the study of one's own scriptures. Today it has the overtone of studying everything that deals with the nature of man.

SVASTIKASAN
The auspicious pose.

TADA
The palm-tree pose.

TADA-NANASKARA
The rocking chair pose.

TALAS
Centers that exist in the thigh bone area, that are related symbolically to the lower nether realms.

TAMAS
One of the three qualities or gunas in nature. It is the psychocosmic principle of inertia. (See *guna*.)

TANMATRA
The five basic principles corresponding to the five sensations such as seeing, hearing, etc. appearing in consciousness, and thus giving rise to the five sense organs: the eyes, the ears, etc. These esoterically correspond to the five subtle states of matter called elements: earth, water, fire, air, and ether.

TANTRA(S)
A text or treatise on yoga which offers methods referred to as kriya yoga, laya yoga, and/or kundalini yoga. In the practice of Kriya Yoga, it should be understood that the technique is always internal and individual.

TANTRA YOGA
The yoga of the union of the male and female principle. In the exoteric tradition, it is called the left-hand method or the 'dark method,' in which physical bodies are utilized. In the esoteric tradition, it is called the right hand method or 'the path of light,' in which these two principles are located inside one's own body or self.

TAPAS
Austerity. The root word means 'to heat up, or make hot.' Thus the connotation is to purify through ardent actions.

TARAKA
Refers to the star seen in the ajna chakra during meditation.

TAT
Means 'That,' and refers to the Reality, also called The Boundless.

TATTVA (TATTWA)
The true state or condition of anything. When applied to substance or matter, it relates to the five ultimate impulses of creation: ether, air, fire, water, and earth. Each of these five tattvas corresponds to a chakra and forms the basis of a loka of the inner and invisible life.

TAT-TVAM-ASI (TATTVAMASI)
This famous watchword means, 'That thou art!' 'THAT' is a word-symbol for the Reality. The reversal of this sentence would be incorrect: 'Thou art that' would lead the student to continue to think of the 'thou' as that which he now thinks himself to be, rather than the truth. 'That' (Reality) is what you really are (although you might have an erroneous notion of what the 'you' really is).

TIRTHA
A yogi who vows to walk from holy place to holy place until the death of his physical body.

TIRTHAS
Important places of spiritual pilgrimage. In the yoga philosophy they are internal places for the mind to walk towards. This produces spiritual cleansing, the removal of karma, and sacred blessings.

TITIKSHA
The acceptance of one's present karmic condition to the degree that there is not even a subconscious antagonism, nor a discontentment, and therefore not even impatience. This is one of the six 'attainments' (shat-sampatti).

TRATAKA
Solar-lunar eye cleansing.

TRETA YUGA
The third yuga. It is three times as long, and three times better than the Kali Yuga.

TRI BANDHA ASAN
The three-lock pose.

TRI BANDHA KUMBHAKA
The three-lock breath.

TRI GUNAS
The three qualities inherent in primordial matter, which are often
called: darkness, fire, and Light.

TRIKONA
The triangle pose.

TRI MURTI
The three manifestations of form:
    Creation by Lord Brahma,
    Sustainment by Lord Vishnu,
    Re-dissolution by Lord Shiva.

TRIPHALA
A medicinal chemical; soap.

TRISHNA
Craving or desire.

TULA
The balance pose.

TURIYA
The fourth state of consciousness reached when one enters into deep
meditation. This deep meditation transcends the workings of thought-
patterns and knowledge (in the general sense). It is a state that cannot be described in terms of the first three states of consciousness:

1. A thought, or
2. Love, or
3. Willing.

Turiya is also considered the fourth state of consciousness beyond
the other three which the average earthling experiences: waking,
dreaming, sleeping.

UBTAN
A medicinal chemical.

UDANA
The vital air existing at the Mercury chakra and concerned with the process of respiration. The color is pale or bluish white. It has a great deal to do with the vitality of the intellect.

UDDI-YANA
The exercising and training of the abdominal muscles.

UDDIYANA BANDHA
A bandha performed by pushing the stomach muscles slightly in and up, repeatedly.

UDJAYA (UJJAYA)
The hissing breath.

UGRASAN
The powerful pose.

UNMANI
A state of trance caused by various yoga practices.

UNMANI SAMBHAVI
When the eyes are held open, but no object is perceived.

UPA-DANA
The unchanging sub-substance of prakriti from which all things are projected or molded.

UPA-RATI
The suspension of all personal desires. Uparati is one of the six attainments (shat-sampatti).

UPADANA DARANA
The most proximate cause of an event, mental, astral or physical.

UPADHI
The distinguishing characteristics or 'marks' of a person or thing.

UPADI
'Things' that hide or cover up the clear seeing of Reality. The Upadis can be dissolved by constant yoga practice and continual renunciation.

UPANISHAD
The ancient mystical texts found at the end of the *Vedas*, containing the direct revelation of Truth by the yogic sages. They are referred to as the Forest Teachings, and are concerned with the deeper, inner meanings of the spiritual life.

The word *Upanishad* is often interpreted as 'sitting at the feet of the Guru.' There are symbolically only 108 Upanishads. But, today, there exist over 200, many of very recent origin.

USAS
The Devi of the Dawn, also known as Daughter of the Sky, as well as Lady of Light. She opens the twin doors of heaven and reveals herself in total splendor.

UTKATA
The squat pose.

UTTANA TAVA
The leg lift pose.

UTTARA BASTI
Genital cleansing.

UTTHITA JAMU SHIRA SAMYUKTA
The head on knee pose.

UTTHITA KUMDHAKA
The twist around waist pose.

UTTHI-TARDHA CHAKRASAN
The half-wheel pose.

VA
(See *bija-mantra*.)

VACHIKA AHIMSA
Verbal non-violence.

VAIRAGYA
Dispassion or renunciation, especially regarding the emotions.

VAISHESHIKA
One of the orthodox schools of philosophy dealing with the principles of analysis of the universe.

VAISHYA
The third of four castes. They are the merchants.

VAJRA
The lightening bolt pose. Also called the zen pose.

VAK
Means 'word' or 'speech.' More accurately, the power of speech generated by the yogi through the practice of yoga.

VAKA
The heron pose.

VAMAN-DHAUTI
Excess water drunk on a full stomach and regurgitated. A cleansing technique.

VARANASI
One of the seven sacred cities of India, considered to be the oldest city on earth. Its other names are Benares and Kashi. It is considered the holiest of the pilgrimage cities. Even today, it remains one of the great centers of learning. It is also preeminently the city of Lord Shiva. Varanasi is likened to the top of the skull, considered to be the center of wisdom which abides in the lotus of the thousand petals.

VARI-SARA DHAUTI
The wind-stomach cleansing technique.

VARUNA (SRI)
One of the earliest Vedic gods, who is extremely similar in character to the Avestian Ahur Masda: the God of Light. Varuna is called The Great Asura. Varuna appears to be the all-encompassing sky, derived from the root *vri*, meaning 'to cover' or 'to encompass.' As one of the adityas, he is associated with celestial order, particularly the regular movement of the Sun and the appearance of dawn. Varuna is also one of the secondary nadis.

VASANA
Most people think it means 'desires.' However, it really refers to the habits and/or tendencies that desires create.

VASHI-KARA
Controlled detachment. It is the fourth stage of sense-withdrawal.

VASTRA DHAUTI
Cloth stomach cleansing.

VASU(S)
The name of a class of devas regarded as atmospheric powers like the rudras, the adityas, the asvins, and the maruts. They are most often associated with Lord Agni and the king of the gods, Lord Indra. They are frequently mentioned in the *Rig Veda,* and are constantly being employed to grant benefits. They were held in great esteem in early Vedic times. The key symbolism is that the Vasus have a special relationship with Lord Indra. They presented him with a magic steed which they fashioned from the Sun. They also form a team which drew Lord Indra's chariot. The Vasus are classified in the Brihad-aranyaka as the High Devas.

VASUDEVA
One of the names of Lord Krishna. Mystically, it is also the name of the Father of Lord Krishna.

VASUKI
The mythical serpent-son of Kadru. He was one of the naga kings. The world is supported on Vasuki's many heads.

VAYA VIYA KUMBHAKA
Balancing-both-chalices-breath.

VAYU
Vayu means 'wind' or its personification, and comes from the root *VA*, meaning 'to blow.' Vayu is used in the sense of wind or air, except in the *Rig Veda* where vayu is said to be the breath of the Spirit. This description has become the basis of much mystical speculation about the vital breath: the pranas.

The vayu, in all its aspects, is regarded as having purifying properties or powers, and therefore as being capable of freeing one from misfortune. Vayu is closely associated with Lord Indra, the king of the devas, who was drawn by a pair of horses, one red and one purple.

VEDANTA
One of the orthodox schools of philosophy dealing with the principle of the speculative knowledge of Reality. A school of philosophy based upon the teaching of the *Vedas*.

VEDAS
The primary Hindu scriptures. The word 'Vedic' refers to these scriptures.

VICHARA
Deep and continual thinking by which knowledge is attained. It also refers to a higher, spontaneous thought process associated with samadhi.

VIDEHA (MAHA-VEDEHA)
Deha means 'body.' V*ideha* means 'bodiless,' and *maha* means 'great.' Therefore, maha-videha means the 'great bodiless state,' which refers to a thinking pattern. When a person thinks of himself as body, or even as mind, he is 'embodied' within that thought. When one does not think of himself as body or mind, he exists in the 'great bodiless state' (of consciousness). If a person can exist without thinking that he is either the body or the mind, that person exists in an excorporeal world, allowing the consciousness to astral travel, and to transcend time in a visional state.

VIDEHA-MUKTI
The doctrine of Liberation at disembodiment. It is the idea that Liberation accompanies and synchronizes with the casting off of the

physical body at the time of 'death.' It is possible to be liberated and also bodiless. It is not, however, possible to obtain Liberation while bodiless. Thus, the need for reincarnation, and the purpose of the earth life.

VIDJNANA
Generally refers to secular knowledge, or intellectual understanding as distinct from wisdom (jnana). However, some people inter-exchange the meanings.

VIDYA
Knowledge.

VIDYA-ADHARA(S)
Spirits that are symbolized in Western tradition as air or aerial spirits, and are known as the bearers of wisdom. They are known to carry either garlands of flowers which symbolize the spiritual victory, or swords which represent wisdom that can cut through ignorance.

VIJNANA
Consciousness; intelligence.

VIJNANA-MAYA-KOSHA
The temporal knowledge sheath. (See *kosha*.)

VIKALPA
Means 'imagination.' It is one of the five types of ideas (vrittis) existing in the lower mind, or chitta.

VILOMA
Counter current nadi breath.

VIPARITA KARANA
The reverse pose.

VIRA-ASAN
The hero pose. Sometimes call the vigorous pose.

VIRAJ (SRI)
Viraj is associated with Purusha by whom all things were engendered: celestial, terrestrial, transcendent and transient. From Purusha, Viraj was born and from Viraj, Purusha was born. Viraj is both feminine

and masculine; thus, in later works he is regarded as secondary to Lord Brahma, who also divided himself into male and female, and then united with the female half and begot the male power, Viraj.

VISAMA VRITTI
Irregular motion breath.

VISH (or VISHAYA)
A type of poison.

VISHNU (LORD)
The Lord of Preservation. He incarnates from age to age for the re-establishment of the Dharma.

VISHNU PURANA
One of the ancient texts of India. The Puranas are 36 in number. There are 18 major Puranas and 18 minor Puranas.

VISHUDDHA
The Mercury chakra existing in the throat area. (See *chakra*.)

VISHVA
This word means, 'the world in its entirety,' or the Cosmos. It stands for the concept that the Entirety in its unfathomed, multidimensional, energetic existence arises from within the infinity of the Absolute, which is ruled by the divine laws of karma.

VISHVADARA
Universal man; the whole collection of embodied and objective individuals, not as a unit but as an allegorical forest. It is also one of the secondary nadis.

VISHVADEVA
This literally means 'all divine' and is a class of minor devas. They are the sons of Sri Mata Vishva, who is the daughter of Daksha.

VISSTRITA PADA
The balancing V-leg stretch.

VITARKA
Obstacles on the Path.

VIVEKA
Discrimination.

VRIKSHASAN
The tree pose, also known as the tripod headstand.

VRISHCHIKA
The scorpion pose.

VRITTI
The word means 'whirlpool.' They are the ideas in the lower mind (chitta). Sri Patanjali states that these vrittis manifest in five main groups:

1. Correct ideas (pramana)
2. Wrong ideas (viparyaya)
3. Fancies (vikalpa)
4. Ideas acquired in sleep (midra)
5. Memories (smriti)

One of the more essential practices in yoga is to continually watch the mind (chitta), and as an idea arises into consciousness, to instantly place it into one of the five groupings.

VYAHRITI
The three mystical utterances at the beginning of the Gayatri Mantra (after the OM): BHU, BHUVA, SVAH. Over and above the deep mystical meaning of these sounds, they exoterically refer to the three realms (lokas) in which the meditation of the mantra will have simultaneous effects.

VYAKTAM
The Unmanifest.

VYANA
This vital breath is described as moving all over the body, and is essential to all the channels. It relates in particular to the Martian and Saturn chakras. Because of this, excessive sexual activity, or even excessive sexual thought appears to deplete the general vyana of the whole body—whereas sexual abstinence intensifies this vital air.
    The color of this vayu is red or pale red. When the body and mind are in unusually good health, this vyana can be seen as extending a

little beyond the physical body and is called the *aura*. When we come into contact with people who have strong vyana, it improves our health and also makes us feel good. This is the basis of the Guru's blessing, when we sit at his feet. When there is an abundance of this vyana, it can be consciously sent to others in need.

VYASA
A great sage who is famous because of his commentary of *Patanjali's Yoga Sutras*.

VYATI-REKA
Inclusive detachment. It is the second stage of sense-withdrawal.

There are no Sanskrit words beginning with the letter 'W.'

There are no Sanskrit words beginning with the letter 'X.'

YA
(See *bija-mantra*.)

YAJNA (YETNA)
Sacrifice. The term does not refer to sacrificial *animals*. The universe, according to yoga, is established upon the concept of sacrifice. Even the Primordial Being sacrificed Itself to establish and maintain the Universe. Thus, the yogi realizes that life is to be seen as a continuous sacrifice. Thus, the inner sacrifice is the dedication of one's self and one's life to a higher purpose: the serving of all life-forms.

YAJNO-PAVITA
The sacred thread of three strings worn over the shoulder and around the chest by Brahmins. When the thread is first put on, the following words are said: 'Put on the Sacred Thread, the holy, the supreme, which came into existence along with Prajapati, which gives long life. Let it give you strength and Light.'

YAKSA(S)
Collective name for mysterious spirits that frequent the earth plane. They can be beneficial or disruptive to one's earth life and/or spiritual life.

YAMA
The practices of the five abstinences from greed, untruth, injury, theft, and sensuality. Through yama, the yogi is at peace with himself, and the world. These abstinences must be practiced in action, speech, as well as in thought.

YAMA, SRI
The Lord of Death.

YAMI
Sri Mata Yami was the sister of Sri Yama, the ruler and the judge of the dead. Yama was considered to be the first man to die. Yami suggested to Yama that their union was essential if the human race was to be perpetuated. He rejected Yami's proposal, thus human beings now no longer perpetuate themselves with the same body.

YAMUNA
The name of an extremely famous river mentioned in the *Rig Veda,*
more commonly called Jamuna (Yamuna). It is symbolically identified with Yami. It descends from the Himalayas and is one of the
great tributaries of the Ganges, which it joins at the holy city of
Allahabad. From this river is derived a holy salve possessing great
spiritual healing properties.

YANODDI-YANA
The flying bird pose.

YANTRA
A mystical diagram that possesses occult energies, which strongly
affect the astral body and the flow of pranic energy. Yantras are charts
to stimulate inner visualization and/or meditation. The greatest of all
the yantras is your horoscope.

YASHASVINI
One of the secondary nadis.

YATA-MANA
Progressive detachment. The first stage of sense-withdrawal.

YOGA
One of the orthodox schools of philosophy dealing with the practice
of attaining union with the Reality. The other five orthodox schools all
use yoga techniques to attain their insight (darshan). The path of yoga,
the discipline of yoga, and the techniques of yoga all lead to Cosmic
Consciousness.
     Yoga means 'union,' and it is that state when your life of action
and thought are in harmony with the very source of your being. Yoga
denotes a psychosomatic relationship, a functioning on the
profoundest level of your unconscious — beyond the limits of thought
and language. It is allowing consciousness to freely flow in the prana
currents that pervade time and space.

YOGA ASAN
The union pose.

YOGA MUDRA
The symbol of yoga.

YOGA-SIDDHI
Internalized abilities to commune with higher states of consciousness within oneself.

YOGI
A man who practices yoga with dedication.

YOGINI
A woman who practices yoga with dedication.

YOGODA
A dynamic tension technique.

YONI
The female principle.

YONI MUDRA
A technique for astralizing consciousness.

YUGA
The world's existence has four ages or periods. The first period called Krita Yuga lasts for 1,728,000 earth-years. The second period called Treta Yuga lasts for 1,296,000 earth years. The third period, Dvapara, lasts for 864,000 earth years. We are currently in the fourth period called Kali Yuga, which lasts for a period of 432,000 earth years. Thus the four yugas total 4,320,000 earth years and constitute a great yuga (maha yuga). Each age, from the highest spiritual Krita, to the lowest, Kali, is reduced by one-fourth, indicating a reduction of the spiritual qualities with which people are born. According to classical Indian thought, Kali Yuga started at the death of Lord Krishna approximately 3,200 B.C.E.

A period of 1,000 maha yugas is known as a *kalpa* and is equivalent to a day in the life of Lord Brahma.

A day is equal to 4,320,000,000 earth years. By the Puranic system, a kalpa is divided into 14 periods, referred to as *manu-avataras*, consisting of 21 maha yugas.

Some of the Puranas state that the Day of Brahma is the daylight time, and therefore, to make up a true symbolic 24-hour day in the Day of Brahma, a night of Brahma must manifest of equivalent time.

The Puranas point out that Brahma lives 100 days or 245,600,000,000 earth years. This is the longest period within the Hindu time scale. This period of time is called a *para*. In the theory of the kalpas, at the completion of one kalpa and its redissolvement, another kalpa begins again, ad infinitum.

In the Krita Yuga, souls are endowed with all four virtues: kindness, devotion, charity, and truth. In this Golden Age, Lord Vishnu came as the avatara of a fish, tortoise, and lion-headed one.

In the Treta Yuga, only three virtues remain: kindness, devotion and charity. Truth gave way to falsehood. In this age, Lord Vishnu came as Rama and Para-surama.

In the third yuga, Dvapara Yuga, people lost one more virtue. Besides having gained falsehood, they acquired hardened hearts, even though they retained the virtues of charity and devotion. In this age, Lord Vishnu came as Lord Krishna.

In the present age, called Kali Yuga, one more virtue is lost, that of devotion. Thus, the only spiritual quality remaining in Kali Yuga is charity. This manifests very weakly in most souls. In this age, the incarnation of Lord Vishnu came as Lord Buddha and will come as Lord Kalki.

There are no Sanskrit words beginning with the letter 'Z.'

OM TAT SAT OM

AN INDEX OF KEY ENGLISH
MYSTICAL TERMS

ABSOLUTE
The ultimate, transcendental (yet eminent) Reality. Referred to as Brahman, Atma, Ishvara. 'It' is suprapersonal, supraconscious, and supramental. It is beyond form and power. This does not imply a void. The yogis call the Absolute, 'Life.' This is why all life is sacred. It is that which is considered as the source of mind and matter, yet cannot be proven by observation. It is knowable, but inexpressible. Most mystical schools refer to It as Life, or Pure-Consciousness, as opposed to the content of consciousness. To know Life, or that Pure-Consciousness, is the goal of yoga.

ABSTINENCE
Disciplining the emotions so there is no wasted energy due to sensual cravings, sexual or otherwise. This is a major method for accumulating and directing the psycho-biological energies towards a deeper spiritual goal. The abstinences can be for various periods of time: one week, one month, one year, etc. Irrevocable abstinence is not for most people.

ACTOR, THE
The metaphor often used by mystical schools. It reminds us that while working at the development of our personalities and our duties, we should not forget that we are the actor, and not the part being played on the stage of life.

ADEPT
A person who totally understands the Path and has awakened from the dream of 'just eating, working, reproducing, and sleeping.'

AGES
(See *yuga*.)

ALLIGATOR, THE
This analogy teaches us that if we are merely living to please our body, we are like a person who is crossing a river by stepping on logs, not knowing they are alligators.

ANIMALS, THE LESSON OF
The lesson of the animals is to understand that we should not be caught in a 'net' by the five senses. These five senses are symbolized by the deer, the elephant, the fish, the moth, and the bee. The deer is lured to his death by soft music made by the hunter. The elephant is caught while rubbing itself against a tree. The moth is brought to its death by its sight, the fish by its taste, and the bee by its sense of smell.

ARTIST, THE
This metaphor teaches the lesson that while striving to paint a picture, the artist is really striving to obtain a given state of consciousness, developing his own inner feelings. When it is seen that the painting is temporary, and that the 'person' is permanent, one can then understand that all work performed is truly for the sake of the Self.

ASTRAL BODY
Also known as the subtle body. Earthlings have three bodies: a gross body, an astral body, and a causal body. The gross or dense body is called sthula upadhi. The subtle or astral body is called sukshma upadhi. The causal body is known as karana upadhi. (*Sharira* is another common word used for body.) *Upadhi* refers to a distinguishing characteristic. These are of four kinds in man:

1. Sanjna -   essential state of being; degree of awakening, or evolutionary status.
2. Gunas -   mind or astral body qualities.
3. Kriya   -   actions done by the gross body.
4. Jata   -   status in life arising from karma.

ATTENTION WITHOUT TENSION
This maxim, 'Full attention without any tension' is the watchword of yoga. In the beginning, in the outer development, force is used. With this, tension develops. However, in the later, inner development, that which was one's best friend (force), becomes one's worst enemy. It is especially true in the practice of meditation.

AWAKENING
The True Awakening is to awaken from the world into the real world, which is just like awakening from a dream state into the world. It produces an expanded horizon of awareness, greater self-awareness, and a greater intensity of being.

BEYOND, THE
This term is used to indicate that state of consciousness that is beyond the field of manifestation. In short, it is consciousness of consciousness, or consciousness of the container, not of the contents of the container.

BODY, THE
Yoga conceives the earthling's body to be a nest of three different bodies: a gross, a subtle, and a supersubtle body. Furthermore, within these bodies is nesting the five sheaths. This nest of eight 'bodies' has at the lowest level the *talas*-body, though most people think the lowest level is the physical body. At the higher level is the causal body. These are generally linked to the concept of the chakras, which are mass-energy converters.

BODY, PERFECTIONS
The *Upanishads* state that the perfections of the body are calmness, good functioning, lightness, good complexion, and slenderness. *The Yoga Sutras* say that they are correct form, mental beauty, strength, and a firm 'well-knitness.' These concepts are important because many Westerners practice neglect of the body, as well as doing those things that are detrimental to it.

BREATH REGULATION
This is gaining control of the life-force by the practice of regulation of the breath, which has to do with the timing of the breathing pattern. In ancient days, the favored unit was 1:4:2, which is to say: inhale for one unit of time, hold for four units of time, and exhale for two units of time. Thus, if a person inhaled for three seconds, he would need to hold for 12 seconds, and exhale for six seconds. Sri Patanjali, however, makes no such ratio. He simply states that the breath should be longer than usual, and also finer or quieter than usual. The result of this longer, quieter (non-strained) breath is that the veils hiding the

Inner Light will diminish and the Light will be seen. All mystics have discovered that altered states of consciousness will manifest as one controls the breathing patterns.

CAUSAL BODY
The causal body is the inner-most vehicle of the person, and also the very first sheath, called the bliss-sheath. It is called 'causal' because it is in this body that the 'ego-maker' causes the whole process of incarnation.

CHARACTER
Good character is stressed over and over again in yoga. The Gita mentions approximately 27 positive character traits which are needed to lead one rapidly towards Liberation. Some of these are: courage, steadiness of mind, peacefulness, non-craving, generosity, studiousness, austerity, humility, renunciation, compassion, gentleness, cleanliness, and forgiveness

CITY OF NINE GATES
This refers to the physical body, which is also called 'the temple of nine gates': two eyes, two ears, two nostrils, two lower openings, and the mouth. This reveals that the mouth is unique among gates because it is not paired like the other gates. It is the symbol of the Supreme Power: energy which flows IN and feeds or kills the body, and words which flow OUT and feed or kill.

CLASSICAL YOGA
The system of yoga derived and developed from Sri Patanjali's *Yoga Sutras*.

CLEANLINESS
A key requirement of students of yoga. Cleanliness is of mind, body, and environment.

CLOUDS AND THE SUN
This metaphor teaches us that the True Self is always shining, however, it can be hidden by the clouds. When hidden, people think that the Sun is not shining. It always shines, even if not seen. The clouds

symbolize the veil which hides consciousness. Thus, all that people see is the content of consciousness.

CONCENTRATION
The forceful, and effortful directing of the mind towards some concept or object. Yoga concentration is doing what we all do automatically when we pay attention to an object. In yoga concentration, however, we do it for a longer period of time, and with more intensity, so that the mind does not wander away from it because of associated ideas or emotions. In yoga, the mind has two major divisions: 1) the lower mind (chitta), and 2) the higher mind (manas). The lower mind is like a shop full of tools: knowledge and memories. The higher mind is like a person who comes to that shop and begins to work with the tools. The goal of practicing concentration is to increase the mind's power of attention, thus producing a secure foundation for the practice of meditation. Yoga concentration markedly differs from ordinary concentration by its depth, duration and purpose.

CONSCIOUSNESS
Consciousness is what we truly are. Some mystics say that it is that which is at the very core of our being, deep within. Consciousness is conscious of both the body and the mind, and the activity of the body and the mind. Therefore, our consciousness is not to be confused with body or mind, or their activities. Consciousness is simply 'knowing' or awareness, and we should not confuse what we are aware of, with that awareness. It is hard for most people to understand that we are consciousness, and that consciousness is conscious of the body and the mind (and their contents and actions), and that both the body and the mind are unconscious! Kriya Yoga endorses that consciousness is both transcendental and mundane. In short, it is ubiquitous or omnipresent.

CONTEMPLATION
This is known by many Westerners as 'rapture' because of the state of bliss that manifests in the state of contemplation. Contemplation follows after the state of meditation has exhausted the entire inventory of ideas. Thus, there can be no continuance of meditation. Thus, a state of contemplation emerges. So it is that contemplation manifests new experiences (beyond the realm of the individual's collected memory). Sri Patanjali mentions the example of the elephant's strength. We can not know what that strength is without experience. And, he says, to know that strength perfectly, we must enter into the very essence of the elephant. Thus, everything in nature will yield up

its secret if we find union with it in contemplation.
Contemplation or samadhi has two major categories:

1. Cognitive contemplation which has an object of thought, feeling or intent, and thus is associated by form(s); and
2. Non-cognitive contemplation which does not have an object of thought, feeling, or intent, and thus is not associated by form. It is an experience. Thus, contemplating on things has one major purpose: to enhance one's own consciousness.

CONTENTMENT
One of the key requirements of success in yoga. (See *santosha*.)

COSMOS, THE
The cosmos is egg-shaped and divided into seven regions, each having seven times seven subdivisions. These regions are divided into four major domains in which deities and other entities dwell.

DANCE OF SHIVA
The Dance of Shiva is symbolical of many things. First, that the deity only plays, He does not work. Second, He dances on a dwarf whose name is 'Man-of-forgetfulness.' Third, that we are to learn to play, i.e., not to take self or life so seriously. Fourth, it is a call to us to remember that His will power is also within us, and thus to re-energize the will to live, the will to adventure, the will to unfoldment, as well as the will to divine fulfillment.

DESIRE-NATURE
The desire-nature is that part of the lower mind concerned with our emotions about objects. These result from our previous pleasures and pains connected with them. They arise because of our opinions and thus attitudes regarding these objects. It is this desire-nature that gives the strength and the glue to the relationship between the object and the mind. (Or is it, the mind and the object?)

DESIRES
Desires are considered to be very adverse and hinder any spiritual and/or mental achievement. To any soul seeking Enlightenment or

happiness, the mind must be directed by intellect and/or intuition, not desires and emotions.

DEVOTION
Devotion is generally thought of as directed to the source of all Goodness and Bounty. In holding this state of devotion, there arises a sense of communion with that Goodness. That sense of Goodness acts as a seed which brings forth events and 'things' which could best be called Good. One needs to understand the true meaning of 'devotion.' Almost all the time, people do things to get things. That is as far away from devotion as one can get. Devotion, like love, is done in and of, and for itself. Unfortunately, people love to get things. People become devotional to get things. If they could only realize that they must do something to get beyond their (limited) self. One approach is to find an object of love, or an ideal worthy of devotion, and then enter into the feeling of devotion. All of this says that we can choose whether we want the 'gifts of God,' or God. The mistake people make is choosing one, and then becoming unhappy or dissatisfied. The solution is to realize that we want the 'gifts' to become happy, however, the pure feeling of devotion IS happiness itself.

DIET
Sri Patanjali does not make any mention of diet, as the Indian culture has already spelled out what should and should not be eaten, and when, and how much. Other texts point out that a diet of bland food which is juicy, with high grade oil, is recommended. Also, the stomach should never be more than half filled with solids, nor more than a quarter filled with liquids: specifically raw milk, butter, rice, barley, honey and various vegetables. Onions and garlic are ordinarily avoided, as are acids, bitter, pungent and salty foods, as well as intoxicants, meat and eggs. The food that the yogi eats should be fresh, nourishing, easily digested, and most importantly, handled and cooked only by souls holding 'good-thoughts.'

DIRECT PERCEPTION
This concept says that a person cannot have realization of Reality, of God, or of the Self by mere inference, nor by the testimony of others. By inference or by testimony one can only have 'knowledge about' Reality, one cannot have knowledge of Reality. Only through mystical practice can one have direct perception of Reality.

DIVINITY
This is a very old word found in many languages. It goes all the way back to Sanskrit and comes from the root *div* which means 'to shine by its own power.' It does not shine by power derived from another source. Thus it is the basis of existence, whether we talk about God, or the divinity within each person. Thus it has been associated with the symbol of the Sun, whereas the Moon (and the planets) shines only with its borrowed light, and so is a symbol of that which is manifested.

DREAMS
Dreams are very important to the mystic because dreams are a source of mental healing, and thus a means of body healing. Dreams are also the gateway to the astral world. Also, dreams are a map of one's unfolding karma (generally of the next few days), which symbolically show the way to soften that karma.

EGO, THE
The ego is the psychological principle whereby a person experiences himself as an individual totally apart from all other beings, and even from the cosmos itself. This wrong awareness is one of the bases of selfishness, and thus of suffering.

EGOTISM
One of the five sources of trouble and hindrance upon the spiritual path.

ELEMENTS.
There are five 'elements', which should not be confused with chemical elements. These are known by the names of earth, water, fire, air and ether. These elements are never found in a pure state. They are always found combined together in various percentages. For example, gross earth is 50% pure earth and 12.5% of each of the other four elements; gross ether has 50% pure ether and 12.5% of each of the other four elements, etc.

ENTHUSIASM
In yoga there should be no stirring up of enthusiasm nor of emotions,

because using this method for re-charging one's 'battery' can delay one's progress by turning one away from the Inner Self. We more often draw upon our reserves, rather than drawing in energy from the macrocosm.

ETHERIC DOUBLE
That portion of the energy sheath which is more material.

EVOLUTION
This is a modern term indicating an advancement of an organism. However, regarding our inner progress, the term 'purification' is preferred over the term 'evolution.' One needs to understand that purification refers to all three bodies, and all five sheaths.

FAITH
In yoga, faith is not mere belief. It is a virtue needed to find something beyond one's own ego-self. Faith does not mean the blind acceptance of illogical concepts. Faith, in yoga, is the belief that life is not hostile to us, and that we can improve our lives. It really means 'confidence' in life and in self. In yoga, faith must be practiced along with vigorousness, memory, understanding and meditation. They all work together, or not at all.

FASTING
Fasting is a major method for purifying the body and the mind. It is also used for controlling and mastering the sense organs. It is used to slow down the motion and the emotions of the mind and body. It thus makes inturning much easier.

FEAR NOT
The first words or symbolic gesture of the Guru to the disciple seeking haven from confusion, difficulty and concerns.

FEELING
This is a technical word, and 'feelings' are not to be confused with 'emotions' as is done in everyday thought. Emotions drive and pull a person towards, or away from some thought or object. Feelings are states of consciousness that have no force or power behind them.

They do not force or pull a person in any direction. Feelings are pure states of awareness (of things, or of how things are), without introducing any emotions into that state of awareness.

FIELD
A term which indicates the whole field of manifestation with all its objects and actions. In yoga, we are to become the 'knower of the field.'

FORCES
In yoga this term is used in several definite ways:
1. The forces of nature.
2. The forces of the astral body.
3. The forces of 'thought-forms.'
4. The forces of entities.

1. Some of the forces of nature are studied by physicists and chemists. Some of the known forces are sound, light, heat, magnetism, etc.

2. The forces of the astral body manifest as vital airs (pranas), kriya, kundalini, shakti, etc.

3. Forces exerted by thought-forms are generated by the mind. However, once generated they become independent entities 'charged' with emotional forces. They are active until they die. Some mystics say they never die. Other say that the thought-forms stay alive by feeding upon any entity that is emotional.

4. Entities are considered forces in and of themselves because of the power or force of the mind.

GOD
Patanjali in his *Yoga Sutras* expresses this concept as 'The Indwelling Reality' (Ishvara), who is a specific Spirit unaffected by any content of consciousness, by time or causation, etc. The yoga theology states that any mystic achieving Enlightenment becomes one with that Reality. Sri Patanjali recommends the chanting of the sacred mantra OM, which symbolically indicates Reality.

GOD, APPROACHING
Four terms are used to express an increasing closeness to God: nearness, similarity, being with, and conjunction. Conjunction is identical to Enlightenment.

HABIT
Most living is done by automatic habit. The yogi strives to change the habit-pattern by means of the techniques of Thinking, Loving, and Willing. The development of these three mental traits is the first process of practicing yoga. This development continues until Intuition unfolds, which brings forth knowledge of the Self and Life.

HABIT-MOLD
A habit-mold or mood is what controls the type and flow of thoughts within a person. By the use of will power there can be a transformation of the lower mind's habit-patterns. All sense organs have their own given habits which can only be transformed from within. It is a very slow process of transformation.

HARMONY
One of the three divine qualities. The other two qualities are 'unity' and 'variety.' A good example of harmony is a healthy body in which all organs are working together for the common good.

HEALING
Healing manifests primarily during sleep and/or meditation in which the astral body and the physical body relate in harmony. It is possible because, at that time, there is a minimum of unbalance of the astral body by emotions and desires. As the harmony between the astral and physical bodies amplifies, the life-forces (the pranas) flow more freely producing a better state of health.

HEALTH
The harmonious interaction of the three 'humors' which is necessary for spiritual advancement, because illness negatively influences one's attitude and attention.

IGNORANCE
Although ignorance is the most common translation of the Sanskrit word *avidya*, a better translation is 'forgetfulness,' because avidya is composed of two words, *a* meaning 'without` and *vidya* meaning 'knowledge.' Thus it has the meaning 'without knowledge', or 'forgetfulness,' because the knowledge is there, but we simply do not remember, we forget.

IMAGES OF THE DEITY
Images, pictures, or statues are commonly used in temples, in the home, and in meditation chambers. These images are not the sources of power, but are reminders of divine power and thus are of benefit.

INCARNATION
An incarnation is primarily caused by the desire for grosser experiences. For most people, it is the desire for grosser pleasures, a desire to relive the past's excitements and thrills. In life there are three stages of experience: perception, enjoyment and attainment. People generally do not become aware of the attainment because they are lost in the pleasure of enjoyment. The conditions associated with any given incarnation are controlled by a person's own karma according to his own thoughts and emotions, and therefore the person's title.

INTUITION
Knowledge that is not obtained by the senses. Thus intuition is a 'direct knowing' brought about by clearing and stilling the mind.

KNOWER, KNOWING AND THE KNOWN
In the process of development in yoga, it is realized that the Knower, the Knowing and that which is Known consists of only one component, not three.

KNOWLEDGE
The base of all knowledge is fourfold: intuition, perception, inference, and reliable testimony. However, 'reliable testimony' somewhat 'begs' the question of its being a base of knowledge.

LIBERATION
Also known as moksha, mukta, or kaivalya. According to Eastern thought, this is the ultimate goal and purpose of life. Liberation involves a release from the objective conditions, which are due to personal desires and actions. These emotions turn into bondage through possessiveness. Patanjali and other sages recommend detachment and meditation as the key means to attain liberation, nirvana, samadhi, or satori: the release of the ego-consciousness with all its limitation. Liberation implies the ending of the 'soul's' rounds of rebirth. It is forgetfulness (ignorance) that is the cause of limitation. Liberation is like awakening from a dream — with its expanding consciousness and greater self-awareness. Liberation from limitation is the final goal of all mystics. Earthlings are limited because they believe the dream that they are the body/mind complex. When they awaken from the 'dream,' they realize they are Life with all Its wonders, mysteries, energies, and marvels.

LIGHT
Some say it is a symbol of Reality, others say it is the Reality. The *Upanishads* say it best: 'The light that shines beyond the heavens and upon the backs of all, is the same light that is within each person.'

LEVITATION
The moving of the astral body up the chakric system and projecting it above and outside of the dense, physical body, whereby you might experience the higher worlds, planes and/or lokas.

MEDITATION

Meditation is a state of consciousness by which the mind is held effortlessly to a selected concept or object. The practice of meditation begins with simple, concrete objects or ideas, and moves on to very complex and abstract objects or ideas. It then moves on to very subtle concepts. The continual practice of meditation makes the mind very powerful and creative on all levels.

MEDITATION-POWERS

Sri Patanjali gives the following list of powers and knowledge arising from the practice of advanced meditation. These are:

    Knowledge of the past and the future.

    Understanding the sounds made by creatures.

    Knowledge of one's past lives.

    Knowledge of the moment of one's death.

    Understanding the meaning of any symbol.

    Gaining clairaudience.

    Gaining clairvoyance.

    Gaining clairsentience.

    Astral projection.

    Kriya projection.

    Power of mind over matter.

(See *occult powers*.)

MEMORIES

One of five classes of ideas which arise in the mindstuff, and which reproduce circumstances, images, impressions and emotions from the past. This is by far the greatest class of thoughts for the average earthling, who spends most of his mental life just reliving past emotions and patterns.

MIND, THE PURITY OF

Purity of the mind brings about a clarity of awareness, as well as an extension or expansion of consciousness. Sri Patanjali suggests deep breathing, along with a positive attitude, including association with the happy, empathy and compassion to the suffering, and joy for the wise.

MORTIFICATION
Mortification is not advocated, not encouraged, and not endorsed by yoga. Yoga advocates and encourages the development and perfection of the physical and mental bodies.

NOT-SELF, THE
Everything in the field of the mind and body, including the mind and body, is referred to as the not-self. All the objects, etc. in the field of life are tools for instructing and teaching the Spirit to awaken, to unfold, and to serve other life-forms.

OBJECT, AN
Everything in the universe is a compound of three things: object, quality and action. Quality and action are the object. However, most people incorrectly conceive that an object has quality and action. These three, object-quality-action (aravya-guna-karma), are forever connected and inseparable. Every object is action; every action is an object. Each thing 'has' action according to its quality and circumstance. For example, it is incorrect to say that acid acts on iron, because iron acts on acid. The law of nature states that for each action, there is an equal and active re-action. Thus, both act on each other according to the quality (guna) and action (karma).

OBSERVANCES
There are five observances which are
1.   Cleanliness of mind and body,
2.   Contentment,
3.   The study of the Higher Self,
4.   Fervent yoga practices, and
5.   Attunement and attentiveness to the indwelling Reality.

With successful practice of the observances, one builds a powerful and protective aura around his physical and astral bodies, protecting them from the negative magnetism of other entities. It also brings about mastery of the mind so that intuition will manifest.

OBSTACLES, THE
The *Yoga Sutras* of Sri Patanjali lists many obstacles to the attaining of samadhi. Some of these are: emotionality, mistaken views, mental disease, unintelligence, indecisiveness, laziness, worldliness, and physical disease. These all have one thing in common: they scatter the mind and the mind-force. Sri Patanjali points out that to overcome these obstacles, the student should practice one truth which becomes the hub of his life, and to which all other factors in his life should be centered around. This means constant practice (of one method), and continual dispassion (towards all things).

OCCULT, THE
The occult, or occultism, is the study and the gathering of knowledge that cannot be gathered by the senses. To be occult means to be 'hidden.' Thus, the *occult* is the gathering of hidden knowledge needed for the climb from the mundane life to the Life Divine.

OCCULT POWERS
There are many, many occult powers. However, generally eight achievements are listed. Yoga does not support aiming for the development of these occult powers. They should come of their own nature and time. If they manifest, they should be used sparingly, and wisely. These powers are: 1) becoming very small or very large, at will; 2) becoming very light or very heavy, at will; 3) fulfilling any desire; 4) obtaining anything; 5) controlling anything; and 6) directing worldly affairs. These are more symbolic than actual.

These groups of powers can be classified into two divisions: The first group deals within the real personality. The second group is the eighth occult power called 'mastery,' or the power to influence worldly affairs in the life of others (or one's self). (See *meditation-powers*.)

OVERSELF, THE
A term which indicates that the fountain of each person's being, and also the root of that person's consciousness, is the True Self. The Sanskrit term is *adhi-atma* (adhyatma).

PAIN
Yoga states that pain is caused by the conjunction of consciousness with that which it 'beholds.' Yoga says that removing pain should not be by breaking the conjunction of seer and object. One should break the pain by gaining occult knowledge and understanding of self and karma. Most pain comes because of karmic attitude. To change the attitude is to lessen the pain. The word 'pain' is really the Sanskrit term *duhkha* which really means 'unsatisfaction,' or 'unsatisfactory.' This means that we cannot find contentment in this world of objects (because of ill-adapted and ill-suited attitudes). It is just like a person who is trying to become satisfied on unnourishing food. He just keeps eating until he dies of overweight and/or a heart attack. What is needed is to change his diet. We all need to change our mental diet.

PATANJALI, SRI
A sage who lived approximately 2,200 years ago. He wrote the *Yoga Sutras*.

PEACE
A state of mind in which there is no internal conflict with thoughts, attitudes, moods, or external factors. A person should be at peace, in the mist of chaos and worldly actions. Whether or not the world is at peace with him, is another story.

PHILOSOPHY, INDIAN
The major Indian systems of philosophy are six in number, and are linked in pairs. They are: Nyaya-Vaisheshika, Sankhya-Yoga, and Mimansa-Vedanta. These are referred to as the orthodox schools, or Darshanas. (See *Darshana*.)

PRAISE AND BLAME
These two emotional forces are the most important in controlling people. The yogi should seek to do everything so that he remains mentally balanced whether being praised or blamed, so these external forces will not control his mind or moods. The yogi does not ignore these forces, he just does not let them control his moods and emotions.

PRAYER
The effort to call upon, and thus put oneself into attunement with, a higher power, and thus participate in higher nourishment and benefit. Generally, prayer is used by people to get something. True prayer is just an attunement, like love. Strength, renewal, and energy is the outcome. Yogis generally use meditation as the key means of attaining these states of consciousness. The key difference is that in meditation one realizes that the powers and blessing lie deep within one's own self, and not within another being.

PUPIL
(See *student*.)

PSYCHOLOGY, YOGA
Yoga psychology in the deepest sense is a psychology of healing. It is aimed at healing the 'soul,' which in turn will heal the mind and thus the body. Yoga therapy is based upon the cleansing of mind and body, along with a transformation of attitudes regarding self, others, and life. This is primarily accomplished by the restoration of everyday consciousness into a more balanced, selfless, and focused consciousness.

QUALITIES
There are three qualities in nature: stability, movement, and order; or darkness, fire, and light; or stability, restlessness or harmony. The qualities are called *gunas*.

QUALITY VERSUS QUANTITY.
In yoga the goal is quality. One little thing done well, is better than a thousand things done poorly. It is the quality of life that is important, not the quantity (length).

REALITY
In Sankhya Yoga there are two Realities. The first is called 'matter'

(prakriti). Sri Patanjali states that matter is real but that matter is constantly changing form. Despite the changes, there is a continuing substance called 'matter.' The second Reality is known as 'consciousness' which does not change form. However, the contents of the physical and mental objects that exist inside that consciousness are also forever changing.

REINCARNATION
The principle of rebirth. Reincarnation is considered essential for universal justice, and for the completion of one's dreams and desires. If a soul's dream is cut off in the middle, this would be unjust.

RELAXATION
The yoga philosophy states that one should be relaxed all the time. Yoga practice makes this possible. The relaxed mind and body can summon up great energies and powers to solve problems and give direction to Life.

RITUAL
Yoga is linked with rituals: mystical, magical and spiritual. Almost all the rituals in yoga are simple and internal.

SACRIFICE
The term 'sacrifice' does not refer to sacrificial subjects, nor to a ceremony. In yoga, it indicates a life principle. In nature, all things and beings nourish and maintain one another. The spiritual way of life is to give freely what one has, for the benefit of the world in which we live. With this in mind, a person sacrifices for the benefit of the home-life, the social-life, and the business-life. This must be done in the right spirit, and with wisdom.

SCRIPTURES, THE
For a Hindu this means the *Vedas* which contain the revelation of the essential Knowledge of Truth. For the yogi this means those texts which contain insights and methods of the realization of God. Basically these texts are the *Yoga Sutras*, the *Gita*, the *Upanishads*, and a host of yoga texts.

SECRECY
Much of yoga is clothed in secrecy. It is not so much that the inner
Teachings are secret, as they are sacred. The higher one climbs with
the Guru, the greater is the sacredness of the Teaching and the methods. Only those who show innate mental qualities of non-emotional-
ity and stealth pass through the Inner Gates.

SELF
The word 'self' has two distinct meanings. 1) The false self which is
formed by thinking that the instruments of the mind and body are the
Self. 2) The Higher or Real Self (Atma, Jiva, Purusha). It is important
to have a good personality so as to easily function in the world. This
gives time and energy for the spiritual goal. However, although the
yogi develops a good personality, he realizes that it is not the True
Self. In some schools, this True Self is given the attributes of 'Being,
Knowing, and Bliss.' Other schools say that It is eternal and stainless.
Yoga states that only by direct insight can one understand or know
that Self. It is knowable, but inexpressible.

SELF, LOWER THE
The lower self has three parts: the physical, the emotional and the
lower-mental. Each of these constitute organisms which have habitual
reactions and instinctive actions resulting from past lives. One of the
goals of yoga is to make this triple lower self properly fortified, physi-
cally, emotionally and mentally, so as to work well in whatever environment it finds itself.

SELF-REALIZATION
The realization of the True Self. However, this is a dangerous term
because it leads many people to believe the ego-self is what is to be
realized. Also, it leads people to think that there is nothing beyond the
self. We are a wave in the ocean of Life, and we should never confuse the wave for the ocean.

SERPENT
A simile is often used to indicate the error of the mind. A person walking along a jungle path at dusk sees a serpent. He becomes fearful.
Upon approaching it closer, however, he sees that it is only a piece of
rope, but the fear still remains for a while.

SERPENT IN A DREAM
The lesson here is that although a serpent is only a dream-snake and

thus unreal, it has the power to awaken one to everyday conscious-ness. In exactly the same way, objects of this world have the power to awaken us to higher states of consciousness.

SOUL
This term has many meanings. It means 'mind,' 'being,' or 'spirit.' However, in yoga, it has only one meaning: the memory track of the Spirit. The Spirit is that which is immortal. The soul is the memory track of that Spirit. When the Spirit 'moves,' it 'experiences.' These collected experiences form the memory track. It is this soul or memory track that is carried by the astral body from incarnation to incarnation, and forms the karmic patterns in each new life.

SPACE
Space, time and motion are three factors of life with which every yogi must deal. First, he must find his space in this life. This means he must find 1) his vocation, and, also, 2) his space for meditation. Most Western yogis have a room set aside solely for meditation.

The yogi then must find his time. He must find: 1) time to study mysticism, and also, 2) time to practice yoga.

Thirdly, he must consider motion or change occurring in the ex-ternal and internal worlds. He must constantly and wisely adjust to these changes.

STAGES OF LIFE
In Indian life there are four stages of life: 1) the learning stage; 2) the householder stage; 3) the preparation for retirement stage; 4) the re-tirement and inturning stage. (Retirement has to do with retirement from active worldly actions, not retirement from spiritual disciplines.) Each of these stages should be one-quarter of a life period. Most Hin-dus conceive that a normal life should be 100 years. Thus each stage lasts 25 years. In reality, each stage lasts approximately 20 years.

STUDENT
A person who is slothful and ignorant is not acceptable as a student. A person who is accepted realizes the difference between perma-nent and temporary values, wishes to remove old habits, and wants to be part of the solution, rather than part of the problem. Other than this, no talent is mandatory.

There are three levels of students. The lowest level student does not even carry out the directions or bidding given by the Guru. The middle level student has to ask for directions and bidding before carrying them out. The highest level student knows the Guru's bidding and fulfills it before being asked.

THAT
'That' symbolically refers to the unmanifested Reality (Nirguna Brahman), which is Reality without form.

TIME
(See *kala*.)

TREASURE, HIDDEN
The lesson of the hidden treasure is that it will not come to us because we call or name it. We must know where the treasure exists, and then we must work or dig for it.

TREE, THE
This is the famous tree, or Ashvattha tree, which is unusual because it has it roots in heaven, and its branches in the world of earthlings. The goal of the yogi is to cut off the roots of this tree which are in heaven. The meaning is that the creation (the branches of the tree) hides the Creator. By cutting off the manifestation or the creation, the yogi can see the Creator of the creation.

UPANISHADS
Certain books which are auxiliary to the *Vedas*. These *Upanishads* deal with the more mystical teachings regarding the nature of Reality, and the relationship of man to that Reality.

VITAL AIRS
The vital airs are also known as the life-forces, the pranas, or the

vayus. These are the forces in nature which vitalize and energize various departments of the mind and body. This is done with the chakras which are mass-energy converters. There are five major vital airs.

WISDOM
The gaining of a special type of knowledge by which, instantaneously, there is a transformation of one's basic attitude towards life, and thus towards all life-forms and self.

WORLDS, THE THREE
This expression refers to the three regions of thought-forms: 1) the body, 2) the emotions, and 3) the lower thinking. The first releases forms produced by actions. The second releases forms produced by emotions. The third releases forms produced by thoughts.

End

Book Releases
NEW
by Goswami Kriyananda

The Laws of Karma:
Deeper Insight to the Esoteric Teachings of Kriya Yoga
Goswami Kriyananda's text on karma clearly and simply explains the laws of cause and effect. This unique book contains many yogic techniques used throughout the ages to remove pain and suffering. It is a must for all who wish to move toward greater happiness in life.
8-1/2 X 5-1/2 , perfectbound, 183 pages. ... $14.95

Intermediate Guide to Meditation
This book is a companion to Goswami Kriyananda's classic text, "Beginner's Guide to Meditation." It provides deep insights and techniques to expand your awareness and bring greater harmony and balance into your life through meditation practice. It is an easy to read text, excellent for the novice and advanced practitioner. *5-1-2 X 8-1/2, perfectbound, 145 pages ... $13.95*

A Yoga Dictionary of Basic Sanskrit Terms
In this book, Goswami Kriyananda has taken a further step to include some major English mystical terms. He feels this basic dictionary will help the student of Yoga gain a deeper understanding of many Sanskrit terms, meeting the needs of the contemporary student, and being helpful to the general reader of yoga literature. He has taken the liberty of dividing the Sanskrit terms to make it easier for the student to pronounce them. *5-1/2 X 8-1/2, perfectbound, 112 pages ... $10.95*

A Dictionary of Basic Astrological Terms
In this dictionary, Goswami Kriyananda has included the most basic astrological terms that will help the beginning or intermediate student gain a deeper insight into astrology. This book is a superb reference work. It is easy to read and one you should keep with you throughout your astrological studies. Goswami Kriyananda has taken complex astrological terms, not only simplifying them for easier understanding, but also adding deeper insight into their meaning.
5-1/2 X 8-1/2, perfectbound, 91 pages ... $10.95

Pathway to God-Consciousness
Goswami Kriyananda first wrote Pathway to God-Consciousness as a home study course for his disciples living far from his ashram. It is composed of 16 lessons or chapters, each with self-help questions, and reveals much of the esoteric science of Kriya Yoga. It gives guidelines and Yogic techniques for the fundamentals of the mystical search: the evolution from Awareness to God-Consciousness or Balanced Self-Awareness. *5-1/2 X 8-1/2, perfectbound, 130 pages ... $9.95*

TO ORDER:
Outside Illinois: (800) 248-0024 - Inside Illinois (773) 342-4600
www.yogakriya.org -- E-mail: kriya@yogakriya.org
SEE ORDER FORM ON BACK PAGE

Meditation

Books and Audiotapes by Goswami Kriyananda

The benefits of meditation are endless....Many of today's health and medical centers are suggesting meditation as a means to regain the ability to concentrate and reduce stress. Learn to improve your health and well-being, restore lost energies, and attain inner peace through meditation practice.

♦ *Beginner's Guide to Meditation* (Book)

This is Goswami Kriyananda's classic text on how, when and why to meditate. It is simple and clear and gives you a variety of meditation techniques to begin your own individual practice. It contains simple stories and analogies to bring ease and enjoyment to learning and practice. This book is an inspirational way to learn the joys and benefits of meditation. *5-1/2 X 8-1/2, perfectbound, 112 pages ... $13.95*

♦ *Beginner's Guide to Meditation - A Talking Book*

(Audiotapes and book) This talking book gives you the opportunity to listen to Goswami Kriyananda's recording of his classic text, *Beginner's Guide to Meditation.* It gives you the option to hear Goswami Kriyananda's voice as he teaches you a variety of simple and gentle meditation techniques. *Four 90-minute audiotapes (also includes the book).*
Introductory Offer ... $29.95

♦ *Beginner's Guide to Meditation - Book and 2-Audiotape Program*

This program gives you the *Beginner's Guide to Meditation* book and two audio tapes: *Meditation Techniques for Inner Peace* which contains five classical meditation techniques, and *Corridors of Stillness*, a gentle 30-minute guided meditation (recorded on both sides of the tapes).
Two 60-minute audiotapes and the book ... $24.95

♦ *Intermediate Guide to Meditation* (Book)

A continuation of *Beginner's Guide to Meditation.* This book includes added techniques and helps you train the mind to move from limited conceptualized thinking and negative emotions to more expanded awareness. It opens up practice to the deeper levels of inturning and meditation practice.
5-1/2 X 8-1/2 paperback, 151 pages ... $13.95

TO ORDER:
Outside Illinois: (800) 248-0024 - Inside Illinois (773) 342-4600
www.yogakriya.org -- E-mail: kriya@yogakriya.org
SEE ORDER FORM ON BACK PAGE